A Guide to
Mental Retardation

A Guide to Mental Retardation

A comprehensive resource for parents, teachers, and helpers who know, love, and care for people with mental retardation at all stages in their lives.

Mark McGarrity

CROSSROAD • NEW YORK

1993

The Crossroad Publishing Company
370 Lexington Avenue, New York, NY 10017

Copyright © 1993 by Mark McGarrity

All rights reserved. No part of this book may be reproduced, stored in a retrieval system, or transmitted, in any form or by any means, electronic, mechanical, photocopying, recording, or otherwise, without the written permission of The Crossroad Publishing Company.

Printed in the United States of America

Library of Congress Cataloging-in-Publication Data

McGarrity, Mark.
    A guide to mental retardation : a comprehensive resource for parents, teachers, and helpers who know, love, and care for people with mental retardation at all stages of their lives / Mark McGarrity.
    p. cm.
    Includes bibliographical references.
    ISBN 0-8245-1274-X
    1. Mentally handicapped—Care—United States—Handbooks, manuals, etc. 2. Mentally handicapped—Services for—United States—Handbooks, manuals, etc. 3. Mental retardation—United States—Handbooks, manuals, etc. I. Title.
HV3006.A4M36   1993
362.3'8'0973—dc20   92-38846
                                                         CIP

Contents

Preface	vii
Introduction: Historical Summary by John Gerdtz	1
Chapter 1 What Is Mental Retardation?	35
Chapter 2 Infancy and Early Childhood	61
Chapter 3 School and the Child with Mental Retardation	89
Chapter 4 Transition into Adulthood	113
Chapter 5 Adult Living	147
Chapter 6 Senior Living	191
Appendix A The Medicaid Waiver	231
Appendix B Excerpts from Public Law	243
Recommended Resources	251
Notes on Individuals Interviewed	255
Bibliography	257
Glossary	265

Preface

A Guide to Mental Retardation is for everyone — parents, teachers, and helping professionals of all kinds — who know or love a person who has mental retardation. I've organized it around the basic life stages, from birth to senior living, in an effort to discover ways to include and integrate people with mental retardation into the "normal" world.

In researching this book I interviewed many people working directly in the field in order to bring their insights and learning to the reader. I spoke with parents about their experiences with their children and with the professionals who work with them. I am especially grateful to the individuals whose observations are cited throughout the book. They graciously shared their expertise, and in a sense they are coauthors on this project. Once again, I thank them. In particular, I would like to thank John Gerdtz for providing the historical review and for his numerous other contributions.

My own background includes the study of psychology, especially community psychology and bringing about change through changing systems. For the past three years I have worked as an Applied Behavioral Sciences Specialist in a large agency serving consumers who display mental retardation.

I hope that when you read this book you will discover more ways that people who are developmentally disabled can be included, integrated, and mainstreamed in schools, the workplace, and community.

This task is vital to their mental health and happiness.

Mark McGarrity

Note: The identities of the people written about in this book have been carefully disguised in accordance with professional standards of confidentiality and in keeping with their rights to privileged communication with the author.

Introduction

Historical Summary

John Gerdtz

Although the clinical term "mental retardation" is less than 100 years old, people with mental retardation have probably been part of human society since the beginning. This summary will give a brief overview of the ideas and situations which contributed to our current understanding of mental retardation, drawing from highlights of the history of mental retardation in the ancient, medieval, Renaissance and Reformation, eighteenth and nineteenth centuries, and developments in the twentieth century.

Readers interested in a more comprehensive analysis and history should consult the two volumes by Scheerenberger (1983, 1987).

Prehistoric and Ancient Period

This period runs from the beginning of human history to the fall of Rome and the destruction of the western Roman Empire (476 A.D.). There are few historical records, so most of the information we have about life during this time comes from archaeology, and also from anthropological studies of similar contemporary hunter and gatherer cultures. In a hunter and gatherer society, infants born with severe handicaps probably did not survive long after birth. Many of these societies also practiced infanticide of unwanted children, and killed those who could no longer hunt or find food for the group. At the same time, there is archaeological evidence (Scheerenberger 1983, 5–6) that some hunter and gatherer groups supported these group members with handicaps, and these handicapped people lived full life spans.

With the development of urban societies in the Near East (Mesopotamia, Babylon, Egypt, and Palestine) and in China by around 3000 B.C., we have the beginning of a written historical record in addition to the archaeological record. In the available records from this period, there are only very oblique and sketchy references to a condition we would recognize as mental retardation. Surviving legal and ethical codes from the period, including the Code of Hammurabi (around 2500 B.C.), and of course the ethical values contained in the Old Testament, do give some protection to those who were weak and helpless in those societies. At the same time, people who were poor, especially those who were slaves, were often completely at the mercy of others. No doubt many people with mental retardation were included in this vulnerable population. The formal study of medicine began during this period in many societies, and there are scattered references in some of the surviving medical texts to medical conditions (for example, epilepsy, hydrocephaly) which are often associated with mental retardation (Scheerenberger 1983).

The second major development in the ancient world was the evolution of the Greek culture and society which generated ideas and philosophies still influential today. Around 1300 B.C. a group of cultures and city states began to form the basis of the Greek culture and society. Many of the most influential figures in the development of Greek philosophy and civilization had little sympathy for those in society who were weak or dependent. In general, the various Greek cultures and societies placed great emphasis on the development of physical and cognitive ability, and the basic virtues of courage, temperance, justice, and wisdom (Scheerenberger 1983). It was common in the various Greek societies through the ancient period to kill or sell into slavery handicapped or unwanted children. Both Plato and Aristotle recommended that only the "best" citizens have children, and that children with any deformity be killed or somehow placed away from regular society because they had no contribution to make to the life of the community (Scheerenberger 1983, 11–12). This ominous view of people with mental retardation and other vulnerable individuals was to keep recurring throughout history and, as we will see, to be held by individuals who had no problem putting it into practice.

Greek philosophers developed much of the foundation for the scientific method of understanding the world, while Hippocrates and other Greek physicians began the systematic observations and theories which form the underpinning of the current practice of medicine. Hippocrates, in his Hippocratic Oath, gave such a clear and elegant view of the physician's ethical responsibility to his or her patients, that it is still considered by many physicians to be relevant today (Scheerenberger 1983).

The Roman Republic, and the later Roman Empire, continued many of the traditions and philosophies of the Greek cultures. Roman society developed around 800 B.C. in Italy and Western Europe, and survived for about 1300 years in the West, and continued until 1453 in the East. Roman attitudes toward children with handicaps were similar to the Greek attitudes, with infanticide of weak or unwanted infants sanctioned, and in some cases encouraged, by the state. A unique characteristic of Roman culture was the power of the father of the family, especially in aristocratic families, over his children. Fathers could, under Roman law, kill, mutilate, or sell into slavery the children living in his household. There are many examples in history of Roman parents using this authority against their children, while there is no doubt that many Roman parents also loved and cared for their sons and daughters (Scheerenberger 1983). There is some archaeological evidence from the excavations at Pompeii that young children with relatively severe physical handicaps were cared for and well treated by their parents. But Roman society, like Greek society, generally had little sympathy and tolerance for the weak and helpless.

As the Roman Empire developed, there is evidence, at various times, of the beginnings of a rather primitive social welfare system. Some basic systems of education, orphanages, and hospitals for the poor, were provided at public expense by some emperors. Some children and adults with mental retardation probably benefited from these programs for the poor, although there are very few historical sources available to help us know what happened to most of the mentally retarded population during Roman times. With the development of the Roman Empire in the East (the Byzantine Empire), there was a continued development of public facilities to care for those who could not care for themselves (Scheerenberger 1983).

4 | A GUIDE TO MENTAL RETARDATION

With the formal adoption of Christianity by the Roman Empire in the fifth century, some of the teachings of the Christian Church became state policy. There is good reason to assume that many of these policies were honored in theory rather than practice, but Church officials strongly condemned infanticide, and these condemnations were written into law. Many of the local churches also established local residences for the sick, poor, and homeless, and these institutions probably served some individuals with mental retardation (Scheerenberger 1983).

Roman physicians also developed some of the foundations for the scientific study of mental retardation and other handicapping conditions. Claudius Galen in the second century was the first to identify the importance of the brain in human functioning and to initiate the study of neurology. Other physicians such as Soranus of Ephesus and Ascelpiades of Prusa, both of the second century A.D., studied the development of infants and children, the problems of childbirth and childhood diseases, and the treatment of mental illness and mental retardation. Both these physicians made recommendations for the proper care of individuals with what we would call mental illness and mental retardation, and these recommendations seem to be both humane and potentially effective to some degree (Scheerenberger 1983).

Perhaps the most lasting legacy of the ancient period were the teachings and ideas of a number of individuals which formed the basis of a number of religions and ethical systems. The ethical and religious teachings of Jesus, based to some extent on the teachings of the ancient Jewish Law, as well as the teachings of Zoroaster in Persia, Buddha in India, Confucius in China, and during the early medieval period, the teachings of Mohammed in the Arab world, all have profound influences on today's world. All of these great teachers developed ethical principles which would require their followers to respect, and help care for, people with mental retardation, and all others who needed help (Scheerenberger 1983, 20–23.

The Medieval World:
From the Fifth to the Sixteenth Century

The world of the Middle Ages was, in many ways, as different and as complex as today's world. In the Middle East, the medieval period marked the spread and development of an Islamic society, which was to eventually overwhelm the remnant of the Roman Empire in the East in 1453. In Western Europe, this period marked the development of a number of societies in which Roman Catholicism was the established church, although there were frequent dissents and revolts against the established church and the various civil authorities. The medieval period was one of cultural, social, and in some cases technological development, while at the same time, life for most people was a constant struggle against pain and disease.

The Role of the Church

The economic and social dislocations that marked the fall of the Roman Empire in the West also seem to have resulted in the abandonment of large numbers of children. In order to care for these children, and for other members of society who could not care for themselves, church authorities founded numerous orphanages and hospitals across Europe. Many of these facilities were based on monasteries and convents, which also provided temporary housing and medical care for the poor and travelers. The quality of these facilities probably varied greatly, but they did form a primitive "social net" for the very poor, and this population probably included significant numbers of people with mental retardation. Some cities and towns also provided housing for the poor and handicapped, and in some cases, paid families to care for those who would otherwise be homeless and unable to care for themselves. Many people with mental retardation who lived in rural communities and villages probably lived at home, and were watched over by family, friends, and neighbors. During the frequent dislocations as a result of plagues and warfare, large numbers of people took to the road to beg, and documents from the medieval period suggest that some of these beggars were probably children and adults with mental retardation (see Scheerenberger 1983, 33, for an example).

These medieval facilities such as hospitals and residences as part of monasteries and other religious houses were, in many ways, the first mental hospitals, or combined residences and treatment facilities. The "treatment" in many of these places, as described in the surviving records, seems primitive and barbaric, but in the

6 | A GUIDE TO MENTAL RETARDATION

context of the times, was no worse than the treatment provided for many other diseases.

The Inquisition

Another development of the medieval period was the Inquisition, an organization devoted to investigating and eliminating dissent from official church teachings, as well as punishing those who rebelled against the civil authorities. The Inquisition varied in effectiveness and intensity from time to time and from place to place, but there was a general social sanction during the medieval period for torturing and killing those perceived as a threat to society. A major "threat" was those who practiced witchcraft who were blamed for all types of disasters and misfortunes. Those hunting down witches during the medieval and later periods often looked at epilepsy and other conditions associated with mental retardation and mental illness as evidence of witchcraft. No doubt many people with mental retardation and mental illness fell victim to the torturers and executioners of the Inquisition. At the same time, there were those, both in the church and in civil society, who argued for the humane treatment of mental retardation and dismissed the notion that persons with mental retardation were possessed by the devil.

The Islamic World

Services for people with mental retardation seemed to be more humane, and better developed, in the Islamic world during the medieval period. The great Arabic physician Avicenna (d. 1037) influenced both the Islamic world and Western Europe. Avicenna studied epilepsy, and knew that injuries to the brain would have specific effects on language and cognition. He recognized different levels of intelligence, and seemed to recognize the condition we know as mental retardation (Scheerenberger 1983). Another great Arab physician and philosopher, Maimonides (d. 1204), not only seemed to recognize mental retardation, but also encouraged the education of those who are mentally retarded (Scheerenberger 1983).

Renaissance, Reformation, and Enlightenment:
From the Sixteenth to the Eighteenth Centuries

In Western Europe, the decline of the medieval period began with the rebirth (Renaissance) of ancient Greek and Roman culture in Italy and then throughout Europe, along with the political development of nations and states, and the growing influence of merchants and traders. While there had been many revolts against the established church and state during the medieval period, it was during the sixteenth century that these revolts became successful with the work of the Reformers such as Luther and Calvin.

The End of the Old Order

The Reformation began a process of profound political and cultural change. The old order, including the rather tattered safety net of monasteries and religious houses, was swept away in many countries. While many of the monasteries and other religious houses had become corrupt and fallen away from the original missions, they did provide a crude "safety net" for the poor, and their destruction did significantly increase the number of beggars and other homeless persons wandering the countryside. A serious political revolt against Henry VIII in England (the Pilgrimage of Grace) was precipitated, in part, by the destruction of the monasteries. In one of the many ironies of the time, the Pilgrimage was crushed, and Henry's throne saved, by an army led by the Duke of Norfolk, a staunch Roman Catholic. A number of destructive wars were fought between Roman Catholic and Protestant nations, as well as civil wars within these nations, which resulted in tremendous devastation and poverty in much of Europe. In addition to warfare, hunger and disease took an enormous toll all over Europe. People were tortured and killed if they were suspected of witchcraft in both Roman Catholic and Protestant nations.

The Religious Reformers

The limited historical evidence available suggests that the reformers John Calvin and Martin Luther had rather negative perceptions toward people with mental retardation. Both men stated, at various times, that those who were mentally retarded were not completely

8 | A GUIDE TO MENTAL RETARDATION

human. Luther, in what was perhaps a flippant or thoughtless comment, recommended that an apparently seriously mentally retarded child who was being troublesome in a village be drowned by the village authorities. While it could be argued that these were common attitudes at the times, it seems that those who heard Luther's comment were shocked and refused to carry out his recommendation (Scheerenberger 1983; Kanner 1964).

Residences and Reformers

During this period, most people with mental retardation probably lived with their families, but those who were abandoned or had no living family, were placed in various hospitals and workhouses. The Poor Laws enacted in England in the reigns of Henry VIII and Elizabeth I, gave local governments the responsibility of paying for the care of those who were homeless or could not care for themselves. Similar programs were developed in other European countries during this period to provide for those who were homeless, mentally ill, and mentally retarded. The quality of care in these facilities, especially during the seventeenth and eighteenth centuries, was horrible, and was perhaps worse than the care during previous centuries. Scheerenberger (1983, 43) quotes figures from French and English hospitals and orphanages that indicate death rates of over 90% for children placed in these facilities. Even taking into account the extremely high infant mortality rate and indeed the low life expectancy for all during this period, these rates were very high. The information left behind by those who visited these hospitals gives us some reasons why the death rate might be so high. Scheerenberger quotes comments from a number of these visitors in the sixteenth, seventeenth, and eighteenth centuries in a number of countries who found the residents in these hospitals in filthy, crowded wards, rarely fed, and sometimes chained for life in dark basements.

There were reformers who tried to improve conditions in a number of countries. In the seventeenth century, the French priest Vincent de Paul (later canonized as St. Vincent de Paul) rejected the concept that people with mental illness or mental retardation were witches, and claimed that those with physical and mental illness have a right to be cared for and protected. Vincent de Paul founded a number of religious organizations whose responsibilities included caring for people with mental retardation and mental illness in a humane fashion. Later reformers include Philipe Pinel, who in the late 1700s reformed the conditions at the Bicêtre Hospital in Paris by taking the residents out of chains, demanding that the staff act in a humane manner toward the residents, and introducing vocational training and other activities at the hospital. William Tyke, a British reformer, founded his Retreat at York, a model residence for people with mental retardation or mental illness, also in the late 1700s. Tuke had been appalled by the conditions in the public and private residential facilities before he founded his own program.

New Theories and a New World

This period was certainly a dark one for people with mental retardation, but the gloom was not total. Philosophers such as Francis Bacon, René Descartes, and John Locke helped develop the scientific method of enquiry which formed the basis of much of the later work in mental retardation, and Locke promoted the possibility of scientific knowledge in the service of a just society. Locke also discussed, quite accurately, some of the differences between mental retardation and mental illness (Scheerenberger 1983, 41). Other philosophers including Rousseau, and the less well-known Pestalozzi and Froebel, made important contributions to the understanding of child development and the process of education.

The European colonization of North and South America began during this period. In the early colonies in the New England area of the United States there were individuals with mental retardation and other handicaps. The small colonial communities emphasized the importance of all individuals being part of a strong family structure, and if a person did not have a family he or she would often be placed with a family who was paid to provide supervision and guidance (Farber 1986). Even in colonial times there were individuals who could not be placed in any family structure, and the colonial societies then developed almshouses, hospitals, and "houses of correction," to care for these people, many of whom were probably mentally retarded. Many of these almshouses were of no better quality than their European versions.

10 | A GUIDE TO MENTAL RETARDATION

Reformers such as Benjamin Rush of Pennsylvania were disgusted with the dirt and brutality of many of the hospitals and almshouses.

The Nineteenth Century

By the beginning of the nineteenth century, the Industrial Revolution was drastically changing work, society, and family life (Farber 1986). In the United States a flourishing industrial economy provided work for men, women, and children, but often under degrading and sometimes dangerous conditions. By 1818, the American Asylum for the Deaf and Dumb in Hartford, Connecticut, developed the first residential and educational program for children with mental retardation (Scheerenberger 1983, 99). This program was the exception. Children and adults with mental retardation who needed services probably were placed in the hospitals and county workhouses along with people who were homeless, those who were mentally ill, chronic alcoholics, and others who were incapable of caring for themselves or were a nuisance to the community. Individuals with mental retardation from wealthy families, in most cases, were probably cared for at home. The only other common alternative to the workhouse or the hospital was the process of "outdoor relief." As described by Scheerenberger (1983, 99–100), this process involved having local governments pay families to care for those who needed care but had no families of their own. This concept goes back to the medieval period in Western Europe, and in the United States families would "bid" to provide a home to individuals who were dependent on the government. There was virtually no monitoring of the care given in these homes, nor were any measures taken to protect vulnerable people from abuse and exploitation. If a county or local government felt that it were serving too many people through the bidding process, the government officials usually fell back on the time-honored procedure of gathering together those in need of services and dumping them in another locality (Scheerenberger 1983).

Programs for the Poor

It is, to some degree, anachronistic to label the hospitals, almshouses, and outdoor relief programs as bad or terrible services. First, the plight of most poor people at the time was horrible, and hunger, disease, filth, and crowding were realities of everyday life for many people, not just those with mental retardation. Second, these were not designed to be good, or even desirable services. The greatest fear of the local authorities was that too many would be attracted to a life supported by the government, so the aim was to make these options as unattractive as possible. At the same time, we have the records of contemporary visitors to the hospitals and almshouses, as well as to some outdoor relief families, and generally these visitors, most of whom were familiar with the conditions of poor families, were often disgusted by what they found.

Scientific Progress

The nineteenth century was a time of enormous scientific progress, and this century marked the beginning of the scientific study of mental retardation. Scientists and physicians in France (Esquirol, Seguin) and in the United Kingdom (Down, Ireland, Duncan and Millard, West) developed classification schemes to assist in the diagnosis of mental retardation, and to distinguish the various levels of severity of the syndrome. Most of these researchers were not only interested in the theoretical aspects of mental retardation. Virtually all the researchers were involved, at one time or another, in directly working with people with mental retardation and their families, and they hoped their work would assist in the development of effective educational programs and humane residential settings for their patients with mental retardation. Some, such as John Down, founded their own residential programs. This work in diagnosis and classification formed the basis of much of the later scientific studies of the measurement of human intelligence (Scheerenberger 1983). There was a growing recognition at this time that mental retardation was different from mental illness, and there were recommendations that separate programs and services be developed for each population.

12 | A GUIDE TO MENTAL RETARDATION

The Pioneers

Many of these pioneers in the identification and classification of mental retardation also developed education programs for children with mental retardation. Itard and Seguin in France (Seguin later emigrated to the United States), and Down and Ireland in the United Kingdom, developed very specific educational and training programs for children with all levels of mental retardation, and these programs emphasized the importance of vocational training so that the students might become as independent as possible as adults. Many of these educational innovators, like Maria Montessori of Italy, were physicians who recognized that educational services rather than medical treatment was the primary need of most persons with mental retardation.

Special Education in Public Schools: Early Beginnings

By 1859 a special day class for children with mental retardation who lived at home was established in Halle, Germany. From the very beginning of the Halle program, some parents objected to the separation of their children with mental retardation from the general school population in public school programs (Sengstock, Magerhans-Hurley, and Sprotte 1990a, 8–9). The German public special education programs were in many ways the pioneers of many of the programs and concepts we now take for granted in special education. By the 1880s the German system developed specialized curricula and instructional techniques, diagnostic and assessment programs, specialized teacher training and certification, and organizations for parents and for professionals involved in the education of students with mental retardation. The German special education programs struggled with the need to integrate children with mental retardation and nonhandicapped students in the public schools, and also developed some public awareness programs to increase understanding of, and compassion for, children and adults with mental retardation (Sengstock et al. 1990a).

The German model of public school special education programs spread rapidly throughout Western Europe. There is also evidence that some of the innovators in the United States were influenced either by the German public special education system or the specialized, state-funded residences for individuals with mental retardation which began in the 1840s (Sengstock et al. 1990a).

In the United States reformers such as Samuel Gridley Howe, Charles Sumner, and Horace Mann managed to secure state funding for public school programs for children with mental retardation in Massachusetts and other states. These programs remained very limited in scope and resources, but they were the first steps in convincing legislators and the public that children with mental retardation could be educated, and that this education was, to some degree, a public responsibility.

By the middle of the century in the United States, the outdoor relief programs, hospitals, and almshouses were struggling to cope with the increasing demands placed on them by a great increase in population, especially through immigration. The costs of these programs had increased greatly, to the dismay of many legislators. In addition, Dorothea Dix traveled across the United States and visited many almshouses and outdoor relief programs. The abuses and inhumane treatment that Dix found and skillfully documented to a number of state governments, beginning with her address to the Massachusetts legislature in 1843, started the trend of state governments developing and funding residential programs for individuals with mental retardation and mental illness. Dix herself was convinced that people with mental retardation would be far better off in large public residences than in local almshouses or even than living with their families (Scheerenberger 1983, 104–107).

There is evidence that a number of men who had been previously diagnosed with mental retardation fought and died in the Civil War, and some were decorated for bravery (Scheerenberger 1983, 117–118). During and after the war, there was a continuation in the efforts to develop residences for children and adults withe mental retardation, with these residences funded by the state governments. These efforts came from a number of sources. Reformers like Howe and Dix saw the terrible conditions in the almshouses and hospitals funded by local governments and recommended the development of specialized residences. Howe had his own small residence for children with mental retardation in Massachusetts, and he found that when the children became adults it was often impossible to either send them back to their families

14 | A GUIDE TO MENTAL RETARDATION

or to expect that they would support themselves in the community. Local government officials welcomed the possibility that the state government would take on the burden of caring for people with mental retardation and mental illness. Finally, a number of theories began to link mental retardation and criminal behavior, and by the 1880s there was a perceived need to protect the general public from the supposedly dangerous behavior of people with mental retardation. This protection was to be provided by isolating the mentally retarded population from the general community in large residential facilities (Scheerenberger 1983).

The idea that people with mental retardation were potentially dangerous began with some relatively innocuous research in the study of individual human differences by scientists like Sir Francis Galton. Galton, a cousin of Charles Darwin, began to study family histories and came to the conclusion that, just as physical characteristics are inherited, so are many intellectual and moral characteristics (Scheerenberger 1983, 64). A number of studies of inheritance, such as Dugdale's study of the "Jukes" family, reinforced the notion that criminal behavior was inherited along with mental retardation in many families. Dugdale himself concluded that most of the criminal behavior he observed seemed to be the result of environment rather than inheritance, but this conclusion was ignored by many who used his work (Scheerenberger 1983). There was also a growing fear and resentment of immigrants at this time, and in 1891 the Immigration Act was changed to prevent those with mental retardation, mental illness, and contagious diseases from emigrating to the United States.

Many of the scientific and popular writings of the late nineteenth and early twentieth centuries are filled with references to people with mental retardation as "criminals," "prostitutes," "parasites," and similar terms. These attitudes spread the idea that most people with mental retardation were born with criminal tendencies, and that the best form of prevention of mental retardation was to have people with retardation isolated from society, and to stop them from having children by any means possible, including forcible sterilization. There were, of course, those who disagreed with this perception of mental retardation, and fought it as vigorously as possible.

The Genesis of the Large Institution

Under the direction of a number of intelligent and forceful administrators in a number of states (Hervey Wilbur and Isaac Kerlin in Pennsylvania, J. B. Richards in New York), a number of large, self-supporting residential programs were developed. These residential programs were no longer short-term educational placements for children before they could be returned home, but lifelong living arrangements for children and adults with all types of mental retardation. The residents of these institutions were expected to work caring for other residents, or to help support the running of the institution in other ways. The mission of the residence was no longer primarily educational but custodial (Scheerenberger 1983). The administration of the residence was continually under pressure from bureaucrats and legislators to have their program as self-supporting as possible, so there was a great emphasis on farming and food production. These activities had the added benefit of providing productive work for most of the residents. Many of the superintendents recommended that residential programs be smaller and located within communities but, with few exceptions, this model was not very popular. The superintendents were generally decent people who did everything they could to make the residence as humane as possible, and to protect the residents against abuse.

Even with the development of these large residential programs in most states, many people with mental retardation were still served in local hospitals or county workhouses. The conditions in these facilities had not improved much even by the end of the century.

By the end of the century the professions of special education and clinical psychology had developed, and a good research base was developing into the nature and causes of mental retardation. Programs to train and certify teachers were also beginning to appear across the country. Many of the characteristics of services we now take for granted, including individual assessment, systematic and concrete methods of instruction, multi-disciplinary teams, services to families, the development of professional associations with an interest in mental retardation, and many others,

16 | A GUIDE TO MENTAL RETARDATION

had their genesis in the last part of the nineteenth century (Scheerenberger 1983, 131–135).

The Twentieth Century

By the beginning of the twentieth century many of the foundations of the modern welfare state were in place, or starting to develop. The concern about the possible genetic inheritance of criminal tendencies, and the supposed relationship between criminal behavior and mental retardation, led to increased development and expansion of large, state-funded, residential facilities. As the residences became more crowded with a variety of people with a number of different handicaps, while the budgets provided were often inadequate, the deficiencies of these residences became more obvious. The superintendents and other administrators were well aware of the problems in their institutions, and in many cases, took considerable pains to correct these problems.

The "Defective Delinquent" and Other Dangers

Both the professional literature and the newspapers of the early twentieth century were full of the problems and dangers of the "defective delinquent," the adolescent boy or girl, often mentally retarded, who was a danger to self and community not only because of his or her behavior but also because of the possibility that the adolescent would have children in the future, and so continue to burden society. Many of the scientists who were instrumental in the development and standardization of the first tests of intelligence (I.Q.) were very interested in the inheritance of character traits and behavior. Scientists such as Henry Goddard, Lewis Terman, and Fred Kuhlmann were all interested in studies of mental retardation, and tracing mental retardation through family histories. Goddard's study of the "Kallikak" family was especially influential after its publication in 1912. Goddard and his researchers investigated the family history of an eight-year-old girl admitted to a residence in New Jersey. Goddard claimed to trace the family history back to a soldier during the Revolutionary War. This soldier had a brief liaison with a "feebleminded girl," and the descendents of this relationship engaged in criminal and immoral behavior for generations, and were likely to be mentally retarded. The same soldier married a "respectable" woman after the War, and the descendants of this marriage were generally respectable. By the time the study was concluded Deborah Kallikak was an attractive young woman in her early twenties who remained in the institution. Goddard was not very impressed with Deborah, basically because of her family history: "a typical illustration of the mentality of the high-grade, evil-minded person, the moron, the delinquent, the kind of girl or woman who fills our reformatories" (quoted in Scheerenberger 1983, 150–151).

There were physicians, psychologists, educators, and others who dismissed Goddard's research on the Kallikaks as biased and unreliable, but the work remained very influential. A number of other studies followed up through the middle of the 1920s. These studies also claimed to demonstrate the joint inheritance of mental retardation and criminal and immoral behavior through a number of generations.

The Eugenics Movement

This concern about heredity resulted in the movement known as eugenics which was popular in the United States and Europe. The eugenics movement attempted to ensure that only those of "good stock" married and had children. Those who, because of disease, handicap, or criminal or deviant behavior, were not fit and healthy members of society should neither marry nor have children. Those who would not refrain from marriage or childbearing should be prevented from doing so by the state. In 1915, in Illinois and soon followed by other states, it was made easier to institutionalize children and adults who were seen to be dangerous to themselves or to society. An increasing number of people were involuntarily placed in institutions, including infants and young children (Scheerenberger 1983). There was also a strong movement to legally prevent the marriage of people who were mentally retarded, and to surgically sterilize, voluntarily or involuntarily, men and women with mental retardation. These sterilization laws were not only to prevent mental retardation; in a number of states prostitutes, drug addicts, and alcoholics could also be sterilized (Scheerenberger 1983, 154–156).

18 | A GUIDE TO MENTAL RETARDATION

Even though there was an increasing number of legal and social sanctions to support the involuntary institutionalization and
sterilization of individuals with mental retardation, the majority of
the mentally retarded population was probably not institutionalized at this time. Many were supported by their families at home.
Others were placed in county poorhouses and work farms, which
survived in many areas well into the 1940s and early 1950s. The
conditions in the work farms for people with mental retardation,
and for anyone else forced to live there, was generally far worse
than the conditions prevailing in most institutions.

The Uses of I.Q.

This period was marked by the development of the I.Q. test, and
the popular adoption of the various tests by schools, the military,
and various government agencies. Many of the developers of the
tests hoped that the diagnosis of mental retardation would be made
easier and more reliable, and that proper services would then be
provided to help the children and adults identified as mentally retarded. As the tests became more widely adopted in the public
schools, I.Q. test scored were used to prevent the enrollment of
children with more severe handicaps in the special education programs in public schools. In the 1920s school districts in Chicago
and other large cities would not admit students with I.Q.s less than
40; the I.Q. level would later be raised to 50. Some other cities, for
example, Cleveland, would only enroll students with low I.Q.
scores in their special education programs. In general, I.Q. scores
were often used to deny public school special education services
for children with severe and profound mental retardation. Parents
of these children were often told to care for the children at home
or send them to an institution (Scheerenberger 1983). Ironically,
many of those responsible for developing I.Q. tests had specifically warned of the dangers of using these tests as a basis for rigid
classification, or as a means of denying services (Scheerenberger
1983, 180–181).

New Programs and New Knowledge

The events during this first thirty years of the century were not
totally negative for people with mental retardation. Physicians

identified many of the toxic agents (lead, mercury) and other substances (alcohol, narcotics) which may contribute to mental retardation in the developing fetus and infant. The effect of child and maternal malnutrition, some infectious diseases, and some biochemical disorders on the development of mental retardation was identified during this period. Public school special education programs and training of teachers continued to expand and develop. Some of the institutions began to investigate educational techniques to educate individuals with severe and profound mental retardation, and to introduce the concept that no person, no matter how severely handicapped, was "uneducable." Some institutions provided educational and outreach services in local communities, and began to develop small residences in local neighborhoods. These programs were not common, but they formed the basis of today's system of community-based services.

Men and women with mental retardation served their country during World War I, as during previous wars, although there were attempts, through I.Q. tests, to prevent men with mental retardation from enlisting in the military. Scheerenberger (1983) mentions the case of a number of men with mental retardation who served in the military, some with distinction, and then were institutionalized on their return home. There was also a growing interest in the systematic study of mental retardation by faculty in many universities and colleges in the United States and Europe. Parent support and advocacy groups, later to grow into the National Association for Retarded Citizens (ARC) began in the early 1930s. The parents were concerned about conditions in the large residential facilities, as well as the lack of proper special education, residential, vocational, and other services in the local communities. Public school special education programs continued to expand, and often included vocational preparation and trips into the community as part of their curricula (Scheerenberger 1983).

The Depression and the Search for Scapegoats

As the miseries of the Depression began to spread across the United States, and then the rest of the industrialized world, from the late 1920s through most of the 1930s, many programs for people with mental retardation were reduced as governments cut funding, or the programs were eliminated entirely. The financial

20 | A GUIDE TO MENTAL RETARDATION

collapse meant that many families could no longer care for a child or adult with mental retardation at home, especially when even minimal support services were cut. There was a flood of requests for admissions to the large state facilities from desperate families. A further ominous occurrence during the Depression was the development of political organizations in many countries seeking scapegoats for the economic misery. There was a general increase in anti-Semitism, and some of this anger was directed toward people with mental retardation and mental illness who were supported by the state in large institutions. This anger was especially felt in Germany, reeling from economic chaos and the defeat after World War I. Popular German books in the 1920s generated resentment of the supposedly large number of institutionalized people living at government expense while so many were hungry and unemployed. These books helped to build public resentment of the state-funded residences, and the books were very biased and inaccurate. Contrary to the popular impression that residents of institutions in Germany were living in luxury, research by British historian Michael Burleigh (1991, 321–322), indicated that about 45,000 residents of these institutions starved to death during World War I, just in the state of Prussia.

New Ideology/Old Ideas

Adding fuel to the fire of this resentment in Germany, as well as in a number of other countries, was ideology of racial superiority made popular by Adolf Hitler and his Nationalist Socialist (Nazi) Party. Hitler summarized his ideology in his book *Mein Kampf* (My Struggle), originally published in 1924. Hitler was obsessed with the notion of a "pure" German race, and he had a very clear idea of how this ideal could be reached. In *Mein Kampf* he wrote: "A prevention of the faculty and opportunity to procreate on the part of the physically degenerate and mentally sick, over a period of only six hundred years, would not only free humanity from an immeasurable misfortune, but would also lead to a recovery which today seems scarcely considerable" (quoted in Scheerenberger 1983, 210).

The horrors of Nazi Germany and the murder of millions of men, women, and children are too well known to be recounted here. Less well known is the systematic murder by the Nazis of almost 100,000 people with mental illness, mental retardation, or other handicapping conditions. As early as 1929 Hitler was speaking publicly of the benefits of "removing" weak and handicapped people from German society (Burleigh 1990). After achieving full political power as Chancellor, Hitler began to put his words into action. By 1933 laws had been passed permitting the involuntary sterilization of individuals with supposedly hereditary diseases, including mental retardation. In the Fall of 1939 Hitler permitted his personal physician, Dr. Brandt, to initiate a program in which certain authorized physicians were permitted to kill infants with a variety of handicaps: the killing was usually by means of lethal injection or starvation. Within a year, over 5,000 infants had been killed, and the program was expanded to children and adolescents with handicaps, and soon after, to adults with mental illness or mental retardation. The program was implemented with the full, and sometimes enthusiastic support, of a number of prominent academic psychiatrists and other physicians (Burleigh 1991). This particular program, known as Aktion T-4 after the street address in Berlin where the headquarters were located, was only one of the Nazi killing programs. SS and Wehrmacht (regular army) troops in Poland, and the occupied regions of the Soviet Union, killed over 10,000 psychiatric patients in residences and asylums. While many children and adults with mental retardation were victims of this mass murder, other victims, as summarized by Michael Burleigh included "forced laborers from the East who had fallen ill, or had breakdowns, their racially undesirable but otherwise healthy newborn children, and the inmates of orphanages and concentration camps for juveniles" (1990, 13). In a grim example of poetic justice, a number of the SS eventually suffered nervous breakdowns, were placed in psychiatric hospitals, and killed along with the other patients (Burleigh 1991).

While many in German society went along with the murders, a few courageously spoke out. Family members protested the "disappearance" and "death from natural causes" of their relatives in institutions and asylums. Count Galen, the Roman Catholic bishop of Münster, publicly denounced the murder campaign, and even tried to take legal action to stop it. Galen had long despised the Nazis, and was marked for death, but was too popular for the Nazis to send to a concentration camp or to kill. His speech in

22 | A GUIDE TO MENTAL RETARDATION

August, 1941, was so effective that the killing campaign was briefly halted.

Special Education under the Nazis

Not all people with mental retardation were marked for death by the Nazis. As we saw previously in this section, Germany developed a system of special education programs in the public schools by the end of the nineteenth century. This system suffered greatly during World War I and the subsequent economic revival of the late 1930s. The Nazis reduced the funding of the special education programs and infiltrated the professional association of German special education teachers. Some leaders of the previous teacher's association, especially Gustav Lesemann, the chairman, were active in assisting the Nazis in taking over the association, and Lesemann was a strong supporter of Aktion T-4 and similar programs (Sengstock et al. 1990b). The public special education programs under the Nazis were responsible for training people with mild mental retardation to perform "useful work," often farm work or simple assembly in factories, as well as arranging for the sterilization of all pupils. Teachers were also asked to assist in the diagnosis of individuals with mental retardation, although their role was always secondary to the role of the state physicians. Pupils in the public school special education system who could not be trained for work, mainly due to the severity of their handicaps, were often sent to the asylums where they were put to death. There is evidence that some special education teachers resisted the efforts of the Nazis, and even helped provide answers to psychological tests in advance to students who were about to be tested. Unfortunately, these efforts were not always successful: teachers provided the answers to standardized I.Q. tests, but the Nazi state physicians used "Form 5A" (an arbitrary and unreliable test) to diagnose mental retardation (Sengstock et al. 1990b).

Sengstock et al. (1990b, 233) quoted from Peukert's social history of the infiltration of Nazism into everyday German life: the Nazis were "purported to be helpful and constructive, yet moved almost apologetically and in passing, to the eradication of those of inferior value." This subtle and skillful approach, backed up by the deadly terror of the Gestapo and SS, meant that public opposition to Nazi policy only came from those who were desperate, or the very brave, or the very foolish.

In reaction to the success of Galen's protest, the Nazis began to intensify their propaganda efforts to justify the sterilization, and sometimes the killing, of people with handicaps or incurable illnesses. The employees of the propaganda machine were intelligent enough to realize that the hard-core Nazi ideology appealed to only a small proportion of the German population. They skillfully, in a number of relatively effective movies, argued that people with handicaps should be removed for a number of humane and economic reasons. The reasons put forward included the argument that most of the handicapped people would be "better off dead" because their lives were full of suffering. Other reasons incorporated the argument that the existence of people with handicaps (especially those with severe handicaps) was a source of suffering for family members or those who had to care for them in homes or institutions. Finally, a powerful argument especially designed for poor and low-income areas: the cost of caring for people with handicaps takes resources away from other government programs in health care, housing, etc. Some of Germany's most talented actors and actresses, scriptwriters, and directors were recruited to work for the propaganda campaign. Prominent physicians vied for the opportunity to provide technical assistance to the propaganda campaign. Some well-known psychiatrists selected certain children and adults in institutions to be temporarily spared from death so that they could be filmed (Burleigh 1990, 15–16). In spite of the protestations at war crimes trials after the war, there was no evidence that any of the important people involved in Aktion T-4, the propaganda campaign or the actual killing, were forced into it against their will.

Aftermath

The murder apparatus developed for Aktion T-4 and similar programs was soon to be expanded and put to work for the systematic murder of Jews, Gypsies, and any others the Nazis considered "undesirable." Some of the major perpetrators of Aktion T-4 were executed after being found guilty of war crimes and crimes against humanity at Nuremburg. Many others escaped with little or no punishment, and some are still alive today. Michael Burleigh

24 | A GUIDE TO MENTAL RETARDATION

(1991) found that one of the physicians most involved in killing infants with severe handicaps later became a prominent academic pediatrician, and that "none of the physicians who worked in the extermination asylums ever served one day of a prison sentence, and many of them have continued to treat patients to the present day" (Burleigh 1990, 16). Most of those involved in creating the movie propaganda justifying the killing went on to successful careers in the West German entertainment industry after the war.

The evil and tragedy of the Nazi Aktion T-4 program are best summarized by two stories from Michael Burleigh's 1990 article. The first story is of a "cheerful and inquisitive" eleven-year-old boy named Horst who lived at the asylum at Gorden. Horst suffered from hydrocephalus and was diagnosed as mentally retarded. He was an active and alert boy who loved to socialize with others and to sing. A Nazi physician reported that Horst would never be able to do "any type of socially valuable activity." Within two months Horst was dead, the cause of death listed as "pneumonia." The second story involved a blurred photograph and the accompanying caption. The photograph is of a young girl with haunted eyes and the caption reads: "Emmi G., diagnosed as a sixteen-year-old in 1935 as being fit for sterilization because of schizophrenic tendencies — murdered at Obrawalde in December 1942" (Burleigh, 1990, 15).

After World War II

The period from the end of World War II in 1945 until the present has seen a tremendous development in services and programs for children and adults with mental retardation. The historical developments during this period have been so immense and complex that they can only be covered in the most general terms here. Those interested in a complete and readable history of this period should see Scheerenberger (1987).

David Braddock (1987, 182–183) estimated that the federal government spent $62 billion on services to people with mental retardation in the fifty years from 1935 to 1985. He also calculated that 53% of this total expenditure has been in the period since 1979.

Historical Summary | 25

Trends from History

Several major trends emerged from the past thirty years of the history of mental retardation, and these trends suggest the major issues to be faces in providing services to people with mental retardation in the future.

(1) Quality of Life vs. Better Off Dead

There has been great progress in the identification and diagnosis of mental retardation over the past thirty years. Improved medical care has results in most people with mental retardation living normal life spans. There are now a number of programs in many areas to serve senior citizens with mental retardation. Most children with mental retardation live with their families and attend local schools. There is a growing network of small residences in local communities for adults with mental retardation, as well as a variety of vocational and other day programs available. Many of the large residential programs have been closed down, or closed to new admissions, while those that remain have improved their services. Programs are available to help families care for their sons or daughters with mental retardation at home, and there is growing evidence that these family support programs can be effective at relatively low cost. Where families cannot care for children at home, many states have developed foster care and adoption programs for children with mental retardation and other handicaps, and these programs also appear to be effective at a reasonable cost. No doubt we have a long way to go; there should also be no doubt that we have come a long way.

Yet, forty-eight years after the death of Hitler there is still a perception that some infants with mental retardation might be better off dead. These attitudes seem to be held by medical and other professionals, the general public, and even by some families of children with disabilities.

The position that infants with mental retardation might be better off dead is not a theoretical position. The killing of infants with handicaps, either through a direct action or, more commonly, through withholding necessary medical treatment or even nutrition, has probably quietly continued to the present day in one place or another. In the 1970s a number of cases came to public attention which results in some heated, and disturbing, discussions. One case was the death by starvation of an infant with Down syndrome in 1971 at a hospital in Maryland. The parents had requested that the infant not receive surgery for an intestinal obstruction, and be left to die; the hospital physicians agreed, and the baby took fifteen days to starve to death (Scheerenberger 1987, 68). There were a number of similar cases, called "Baby Doe" cases, during the 1970s. Surveys of pediatricians and other physicians, as well as a Gallup Poll survey in 1983, found small but significant majorities in favor of letting infants with handicaps die if that was the request of the parents. There was a disturbing correlation between the arguments in favor of letting these babies die (it is really in their best interest, the family has suffered enough, the cost of care is so high...) in the 1970s and the arguments of Hitler and the other Nazi ideologues. What was even more disturbing was the easy acceptance of these arguments by many who were prominent in the civil rights movement and loud in their denunciations of all forms of oppression. Nat Hentoff, a journalist for the *Village Voice* newspaper in New York, wrote a number of articles in 1983 and 1984 challenging the popular acceptance of death for infants with handicaps, and the titles of his articles on this topic are significant; "The Baby Who Was Starved to Death for His Own Good" (December 13, 1983), and "Troublemaking Babies and Pious Liberals" (January 3, 1984).

Others, in addition to Hentoff, spoke out against the easy acceptance of death for infants with handicaps. Columnist George Will, at the opposite end of the political spectrum from Nat Hentoff and the parent of a child with Down syndrome, wrote a number of effective articles on the topic. The Association for Retarded Citizens (ARC), the American Association on Mental Retardation (AAMR), and the Association for Persons with Severe Handicaps (TASH), all issued statements and policy papers opposing the withholding of necessary medical treatment and nutrition from infants with handicaps.

The attitude that the mentally retarded are better off dead is not confined to newborns and infants with handicaps. The author of a recent article in the "My Turn" section of *Newsweek* (Lyle 1992) argued that it would be more merciful to put to death an adult man with severe handicaps and behavior problems. Many of the arguments Lyle used in favor of her position (death is more merciful and the cost of care is so expensive) were exactly the same arguments advanced by the Nazi propaganda machine.

The most depressing aspect of the controversy was the apparent ignorance of mental retardation, and the lack of recognition of the potential for growth and development of every person with mental retardation, of many of those who recommend death. The lack of concern from many prominent in the civil rights movement was also troubling. The advocacy work of the parents in the ARC and other advocacy groups which resulted in the development of services for people with mental retardation, was inspired by the teachings and actions of the great leaders of the civil rights movement. Those who stand by complacently while people with a certain label fall into the category of "not worth keeping" should study history; the "better off dead" category has a way of expanding to cover many other groups once it is established and respectable.

It is hard to think of a more important, or more basic, issue of human rights than the right to basic medical care and nutrition as infants. Other rights become irrelevant if people with mental retardation are not likely to live through infancy because of a diagnostic label.

Another much less dramatic example of not recognizing the worth and dignity of people with mental retardation is found in public opposition to the establishment of small community residences in various neighborhoods. This opposition usually comes from fear and ignorance rather than a specific bias against people with mental retardation and other handicaps. Even though this opposition has been intense in places, it seems that in general once the residence is established, the neighborhood opposition usually diminishes significantly. As more adults with mental retardation move from large institutions to small residences, and as residences open up to care for those who were never in institutions, I believe that most members of the public will take for granted that these adults live and work in their local communities.

The need to educate the public about mental retardation, and to demonstrate how appropriate services benefit not only the person with mental retardation, but also his or her family as well as the community in general, will continue long into the future. We must also be cautious about those in our society, some in positions of authority and power, who are willing to condone, or actually

28 | A GUIDE TO MENTAL RETARDATION

participate in, the killing of the most vulnerable members of our community. History tells us that this type of killing is often justified as a service to the family, or to society, or even to the victim. There is no need to be obsessed with this danger, but at the same time, we should never forget how easily and quickly this kind of killing can become acceptable.

(2) Rights and Responsibilities

During the past thirty years, many court decisions and much state and federal legislation have been dedicated to establishing the rights of children and adults with mental retardation. Much of this has been in response to years of neglect and abuse. Courts in a number of states have ordered large residential facilities closed or significantly improved, and have struck down zoning ordinances and other laws which prevented the establishment of small community residences for children and adults with mental retardation. Federal legislation such as Public Law 94–142 (P.L. 94–142) passed in 1975 guarantees a free, appropriate public education for most children with mental retardation. More recent legislation, P.L. 99–457, extends this right to education to toddlers and preschool children with mental retardation. Adults with mental retardation have the right to marry and bear children, and to be free from coercion and abuse. Each state has a Protection and Advocacy Agency which acts to protect the rights of individuals with mental retardation and other handicaps. There has also been considerable progress in enabling parents to participate in the educational planning for their children in the special education system, as well as participation in planning programs for adult family members with mental retardation.

The goal of protective legislation, policy, and court mandates is to enhance the independence and dignity of people with mental retardation. While there are still many problems, the legislation and policies have moved us closer to achieving this goal. At the same time, as in many other areas, a "rights and advocacy" bureaucracy has developed, and with this bureaucracy comes a thicket of policies and procedures. Most advocates do a necessary and thankless job, but others can be unyielding in the implementation of relatively trivial policies and regulations. There is a more basic problem than the inevitable problems which are associated with any bureaucracy. The basic problem is: if you have rights, do you also have obligations?

The rights of people with mental retardation are clearly spelled out in many state and federal policies. There is now a trend by some, including some advocates, to question whether some obligations should also accompany the list of rights. Many advocates are uncomfortable even discussing the question, arguing that most people with mental retardation still do not have the opportunity to exercise the rights they are now, theoretically, given. I think there is good reason to discuss the question of obligations even though the battle for full human rights for people with mental retardation has not yet been won. It seems to me unless there is at least some acknowledgement of obligations to accompany rights, then people with mental retardation will always be seen as dependent, and will never attain the goals of independence and full community acceptance. There is a danger that the discussion of obligations will divert us from the need to maintain the hard-won progress on rights that we have now achieved, but I do not believe that this has to be the result. I expect increasing, and heated, discussions of this issue in the future.

(3) Family Members as Advocates and the Rise of Self-Advocates

The current system of services for children and adults with mental retardation exists because of the efforts of families through the Association for Retarded Citizens and other advocacy groups. While the work of sympathetic scientists, professionals, and politicians helped this advocacy effort, there can be no doubt that important legislation like P.L. 94–142 would not have been passed without the efforts of the families. Many groups are now advocating for and helping to develop support services for families, a group of services that has been neglected in the past. Even today, I do not think that most professionals in the field of mental retardation would dispute that families are still far more effective advocates for services than professionals. This is the way it should be. Professionals can, and do, choose to leave the field of mental retardation. Families can never escape dealing with this issue, one way or another.

In the past fifteen to twenty years there has been a movement toward self-advocacy among some adolescents and adults with

30 | A GUIDE TO MENTAL RETARDATION

mental retardation. Rather than have families, advocates, or professionals speak for them, these men and women want to speak for themselves. This is a healthy trend, and the self-advocates have joined families and other advocates in pressing for essential services for people with mental retardation. The self-advocacy movement is in its infancy, and has had its successes and failures like any movement, but I expect that self-advocates will be an important factor in the mental retardation service system in the future.

There is a danger when discussing families in assuming that families of people with mental retardation have the same desires, needs, or opinions as other families in a similar situation. While there may be similarities, each family has individual needs and opinions. There have been significant disagreements over a number of issues in mental retardation, and active, involved, and intelligent family members have been found on both sides of the issues. There is also a potential for conflict between between families and self-advocates. The best interests of the family and of the family member with mental retardation will not always coincide, but these conflicts are not unique to families with a son or daughter with mental retardation. Honest disagreement and discussion is healthy in that it helps remind the professionals, as well as the families, that families are unique in many ways, and that we must be both careful and sparing in our generalizations about families.

*(4) Can You Obtain Special Services
and Still Be Part of the Community?*

Throughout history there has been a dual struggle by those who have tried to develop services for people with mental retardation. One struggle has been to develop those specialized services which are more likely to benefit people with mental retardation. The other struggle has been to fully integrate people with mental retardation fully into the regular life of the local community. After a long history of encouraging the development of specialized programs and services, and of trying to distinguish mental retardation from mental illness and other handicapping conditions, a separate service system began to emerge for people with mental retardation. This separate system had many problems, and as far back as the eighteenth and nineteenth centuries (even before that in some cases), it was noted that people with mental retardation seemed to do well in their local communities if they had the proper support and training.

In the 1970s Wolf Wolfensberger and other advocates developed what they called the "Principle of Normalization." This principle basically recommended that services for people with mental retardation be structured as closely as possible to the everyday lives of ordinary people in the regular community of the same chronological age. In other words, programs for adults should be based on the lifestyle of adults in the local community, and this should also apply to programs for children. Wolfensberger was adamant that he was not advocating that support systems for people with mental retardation should be withdrawn, and he wanted this principle to be implemented according to the needs of each individual. He was dismayed when the Principle of Normalization became a bureaucratic tool, or was applied in the same way to all individuals with mental retardation (Scheerenberger 1987).

The tension between the need for specialized services and the benefits of full community integration is a healthy one. Professionals and families have been challenged to be creative in providing the services that most people with mental retardation need in a way that helps them become, as much as possible, a member of the local community. Even an optimistic view would suggest that we have failed about as much as we have succeeded in attaining these two goals. There have been battles raging among certain professionals who demand either totally separate programs, or programs that are so integrated that there are few or no support services. The battle has been waged with much hot air and furious rhetoric, but the important battle is to reconcile these seemingly conflicting goals, and take into account the unique needs of each individual, while developing a stable service system. No doubt there struggles will continue, but even if we come close to achieving the goal, it will be worth it.

(5) How Do We Provide Services for All?

As this is being written, the United States, and much of the world is facing a prolonged and difficult economic recession. Unemployment is rising, tax collections are falling, and the national debt is

32 | A GUIDE TO MENTAL RETARDATION

higher than it has even been in history. Federal, state, and local governments are cutting services as the demand for these services increases. Those with long memories, or those who read history, will remember how the Great Depression cut the heart out of some very promising special education and other programs for people with mental retardation. Federal expenditures on mental retardation and other developmental disabilities, expressed as a percentage of Gross National Product (GNP), have reached a plateau (Braddock 1987). We are also learning that high expenditures do not guarantee quality programs for people with mental retardation. There seems to be some public resentment of the cost of special education services while educational services for non-handicapped children are being cut. We still know relatively little about the effectiveness of some programs for people with mental retardation, although it is clear that the most expensive programs are not necessarily the most effective or most efficient. Much of the federal and state expenditures on mental retardation are still mainly directed to a relatively small proportion of the population diagnosed as mentally retarded (Braddock 1987).

But I do not think there is reason to despair. Advocates have been able to block some budget cuts in state and federal programs. There is room to redirect some of the current expenditures to programs which will effectively serve more people with mental retardation. Research is continuing on the effectiveness of a variety of programs, and many program have demonstrated their effectiveness. There is now good evidence that vocational programs such as supported employment for adults with mental retardation not only are economically efficient, but can result in a net savings for the taxpayer (see for example, Hill 1988). It is reasonable to expect that there will be battles over limited resources, and potential and actual budget cuts for programs for people with mental retardation. It is the responsibility of families and other advocates to make the case that children and adults with mental retardation have the right to appropriate services. It will be the responsibility of professionals and others providing services to demonstrate that their services are not only effective in that they benefit the people served, but also that these services make the most efficient and responsible use of public funds.

A continuing challenge will be in the provision of services to adults with mental retardation. Children with mental retardation are guaranteed a free, appropriate public education. While there are still many problems with the education provided, this legislation has benefited most children with mental retardation. Children grow to be adults and there is no similar commitment to services for adults with mental retardation. It is not uncommon for a young man or woman with mental retardation to finish a high school special education program and to find there are no adult programs available. This often results in the loss of skills and means that the special education provided during the school years has been essentially wasted.

There is now considerable advocacy focused on the need for programs for adults. I think it is important that the advocacy highlight the special needs of the adults with mental retardation but, in addition, note the contribution that workers with mental retardation can make to the economic growth and development of their communities and of the nation. Not developing productive activities for adults with mental retardation is a waste of "human capital," and the effective training and support of all workers and potential workers is an important factor in achieving long-term economic growth (Koretz 1992).

(6) The Experts Speak

Experts, or those who study and try to understand the phenomenon of mental retardation in a systematic way, have been with us for centuries. These experts have been valuable in developing and promoting many new and innovative approaches to improving the lives of children and adults with mental retardation.

A real problem develops when the expert becomes so taken with an idea or theory that he or she becomes an ideologue. There are such ideologues in the field of mental retardation — they can be recognized by a single-minded approach to situations, with little or no ability to change according to the needs of particular individuals or circumstances. The best way to identify an ideologue is to see how he or she deals with those with differing opinions. Most ideologues take disagreement as a personal affront, and if in a position of authority, will take steps to prevent the airing of opposing viewpoints. Ideologues should not be confused with those who have strong values and opinions. Many people with

34 | A GUIDE TO MENTAL RETARDATION

strong opinions present their ideas forcefully, but welcome the open exchange of ideas and opinions.

The reason this issue is important is that some organizations in the field of mental retardation have taken strong, and generally reasonable, positions on many issues. On some basic issues, such as the matters of life and death, and the worth of every person with mental retardation, there can be no compromise. Some other issues lend themselves to further discussion and clarification. Unfortunately, some of the organizations will not tolerate even the airing of dissenting opinions on the less important issues. The danger here is the assumption that a theory or expert opinion is the "final word" in services or programs for people with mental retardation. Those familiar with the history of mental retardation will be skeptical of this approach: there have been many "final words" in history that have later been revised or abandoned. This is not an argument that organizations should not have strong opinions or values. The words of Sir Winston Churchill are relevant here: "An open mind eventually becomes an empty one." But we can stand by our values and ideals and even make them stronger by encouraging the free exchange of opinions. History tells us that we should also be respectful, but reasonably skeptical, of the ideas of experts.

In their suggestions for the uses of history in making decisions, Neustadt and May (1986) emphasize the importance of policymakers identifying *continuities* between current events and historical events. In the history of mental retardation we have seen the birth of many ideas, the death of many ideas, and the resurrection of some of these ideas in modern times. But history also teaches us that we must also be ready for new and totally unexpected challenges. An important lesson of history is that "continuity is not all. Human experience also includes discontinuity — sudden, sharp, and hard to foresee, if foreseeable at all" (Neustadt and May 1986, 263).

John Gerdtz *is Associate Professor of Psychiatry and Social Services, Emory University School of Medicine, Atlanta, Georgia.*

1

What Is Mental Retardation?

"What does it feel like to be mentally retarded?
Only those who are retarded really know."

Until recently, not much was understood about mental retardation, only that it limited many individuals from living a fully independent life. In the past few decades, insights into causes have been revealed, preventative interventions suggested, and treatment created to assist mentally retarded individuals to reach their full potential. Counseling techniques also have been adapted for these persons with special needs and capabilities.

While services in general have improved, mental retardation is still misunderstood by many, especially those who have never known an individual who was mentally retarded. Even people who work in the field may have different levels of understanding regarding the population with which they work, for example, depending on the type of service they provide.

While many people may come to know an individual with a disability by chance, those persons who are the most surprised and least prepared are the parents of a newborn with special needs.

A Personal Story: Steven

Out of Their Hands: "When our son was born," recalls Mike, telling how he and his wife discovered their child had Down syndrome, "Steven was placed in an oxygen tent for the night

36 | A GUIDE TO MENTAL RETARDATION

because it took his lungs a little time to be fully operational — which wasn't really related to his diagnosis of Down syndrome.

"The next morning, we were given the message that the hospital wanted to make sure that everything was fine, and they were recommending that he be flown to an advanced care hospital. We were surprised, but immediately agreed. And so, while he was being flown, we drove.

"Upon entering the Intensive Care Unit, the doctor, while reporting that Steven was healthy, said that there was a question as to whether he had Down syndrome. It had been a full day since my son was born, and this was the first medical information we had been given.

"In retrospect, the midwife who delivered Steven — speaking somewhat casually and days later — said that he looked different from what she thought he should look like. Down syndrome babies, even at birth, often *are* identifiable by some physical characteristics. The layout of their facial features often identifies the possibility, after which other characteristics can be confirmed.

"The midwife did not say anything to us about the question of Down Syndrome on the day Steven was born, but wrote a note in the chart. We discovered later that the pediatrician acted more on this information to have Steven flown to the medical center than for any concern about oxygen or Steven's lungs."

Reasons for Medical Attention: Only in retrospect can the father understand the infant's need for medical attention. Instead, the father may feel lost in a world of professionals and medical jargon. For example, Mike explains that "there is a high incidence of significant heart problems in Down syndrome babies that requires open-heart surgery. . . . So, there is medical reason for a full medical workup if the diagnosis does turn out to be Down syndrome.

"Also, generally speaking, people who work with high-need babies probably are more able to do the diagnosis quickly. And at the medical center, there are some neonatologists who have years of experience working with Down syndrome babies."

Full Evaluation: Mike discovered that even specialists, despite their training, can err. "The man who did the intake with us,

What Is Mental Retardation? | 37

a neonatologist, said, 'I really don't think your son has Down syndrome, but we'll look for it.' So, Steven stayed for three days.

"I knew the next day, by looking at Steven, that he had Down syndrome, although the medical staff said that they weren't sure — they thought many of his features were not revealing. They said, 'Until you do a chromosome test you don't know for sure, and that takes two weeks.' "

Surreal Devastation: The dream of having a healthy baby does not always come true. Eight years later, Mike and his wife still have not forgotten their feelings when their dream of a healthy firstborn was shattered. "I hadn't had any sleep to speak of in the night. . . . After a 9:40 P.M. birth, my wife had been taken out of the birthing bed, and eight hours later we were in 85° heat driving. The baby had been flown up ahead of us. I was extremely disoriented. It's all really quite surreal to have your baby flown away in a helicopter, have to get up out of a hospital bed and drive for eight hours. We didn't know what we were going to do.

"The doctor's comment about our baby possibly having Down syndrome, after what we already had been through, just added to our sense of surreal devastation. It was almost disbelief — or not really disbelief; as soon as you hear it, it sort of just goes through your body.

"I guess my thought was . . . this isn't really true. This isn't happening to me. This only happens to other people.

"I was also very concerned for Julie, my wife. I mean, I didn't give birth to the baby. She's the one who hadn't recovered yet. I was trying to figure out how to take care of her throughout the ordeal."

A Personal Story: Mark

Discovery: The details may be different, but the feelings and questions raised by the expecting couple share many themes. As another father, Al, reports: "When my son was born, ten years ago, we had a lot of questions — we weren't prepared. . . . We asked the doctor. We asked the hospital."

38 | A GUIDE TO MENTAL RETARDATION

Questions about Help: "Even when we came home from the hospital, we had a lot of questions that were unanswerable. What do we do now? Where do we go? What does this baby need?"

To most of these questions, there were suggestions. "Somebody in the hospital had mentioned that there was an infant/parent program at one of the local agencies that we should check out. Infant stimulation was something new, and supposedly very beneficial for kids with Down syndrome. So, over the next several weeks and months, we made phone calls.

"Finally we found out that there was an infant/parent program. We called them and were placed on their list. When Mark was about three or four months old, we began to bring him there a couple times a week for infant stimulation. This involved physical therapy, occupational therapy. . . . When he was a little older, speech therapy began."

These parents began their education concerning the special needs of their developmentally handicapped child as they gathered information in response to their questions and concerns.

In the above cases, we see parents who have been caught by surprise. Their initial feelings, over time, have changed form — from surprise and shock, to an acceptance of the situation, and later to deciding upon, and following through with, a means of action.

Part of this healing process — if we may call it this — is made possible by information and education.

What Is Mental Retardation?

In contemporary slang, we have all heard the labels "retard," "moron," or "imbecile" used to describe a person who is not capable of successfully carrying out the simplest task. Many people do not realize, however, that these labels have been used throughout history to describe the condition known as mental retardation. In fact, the terms "moron," "cretin," and "imbecile" were once used by professionals to distinguish the various types of mental retardation.

Characteristics of Mental Retardation: Mental retardation is not a disease or a physical illness. It is generally described as a "behavioral syndrome." In other words, people diagnosed as mentally retarded consistently behave in certain ways which are different from the behavior of individuals not labeled as mentally retarded.

The following are some of the important characteristics of mental retardation:

1. Mental retardation is identified and diagnosed during a person's developmental period.

In general, mental retardation is diagnosed during childhood or adolescence. Most definitions require a diagnosis before the age of eighteen, while some permit a diagnosis before the age of twenty-two. However, mental retardation does not suddenly occur in a person's life, but has been present, in many cases, since birth.

If a child is born with a genetic syndrome associated with mental retardation (such as Down syndrome), it may be possible to diagnose mental retardation before the age of three. But otherwise, it is difficult or impossible to accurately diagnose mental retardation before a child is around three years old. "The Bayley Scale is one example of a measurement used for young children," one school psychologist explains. "It is basically a checklist of behaviors: You get a Motor Development Index, a Mental Development Index, and so on. In this way we can get an idea of where the child is functioning in the motor and cognitive areas: Does the baby make sounds? turn his or her head toward light? respond to other people? actively explore his or her environment?"

2. Mental retardation involves significant and prolonged difficulties and deficits in a person's ability to think and reason.

A person with mental retardation will not be able to think, use and understand language, or make use of abstract concepts with the same degree of skill and ability as others. This type of ability is usually measured through a psychological test which produces the score known as the Intelligence Quotient (I.Q.). People who are diagnosed to have mental retardation usually have I.Q. scores of 69 or less, with 100 being the average score for people the same age in that society.

40 | A GUIDE TO MENTAL RETARDATION

3. Mental retardation involves severe and prolonged difficulties and deficits in a person's adaptive behavior.

Adaptive behavior refers to those skills which enable us to function as members of our society, and live up to the demands of independent living. Adaptive behavior includes very basic skills such as the ability to dress, eat, and maintain personal hygiene independently. More sophisticated skills involve getting along with others, communicating effectively, earning a living, solving problems, and getting around the community.

4. A mental retardation diagnosis implies a condition that will continue for an indefinite period.

Some people may temporarily lose their cognitive and adaptive behavior skills as the result of an accident, illness, or even extreme stress: individuals in this situation would not be considered mentally retarded even though they meet the criteria discussed above. An accurate diagnosis of mental retardation requires a strong probability that the handicapping condition will continue for an indefinite period.

Diagnosis

It is important to keep in mind that an accurate diagnosis of mental retardation considers prolonged and significant difficulties in two areas during the developmental period: deficit in thinking and reasoning, and deficit in adaptive behavior. *Mental retardation should never be diagnosed on the basis of an I.Q. score alone.*

This diagnosis is often the result of testing and observation over a considerable period of time. There is no blood test, x-ray, or other medical device which, used alone, can diagnose mental retardation. However, medical and physical tests may be used to diagnose some of the genetic and medical conditions usually associated with the condition, but these tests cannot give a conclusive diagnosis of retardation.

Who Determines the Diagnosis: The diagnosis is usually made by a psychiatrist or licensed psychologist, and draws upon information provided by family members, teachers and other professionals, and by the individual being evaluated.

"What is nice about working at my program," one school psychologist shared, "is that there is a team effort. I may do a psychological evaluation. The speech therapist assesses speech and language. The physical therapist does a physical evaluation, and the early intervention teacher gives input as well.

"All together, this team can uncover a fairly accurate picture. And most likely our reports support each other findings. If they don't, then we talk about any discrepancies."

But not everyone feels comfortable making the diagnosis of mental retardation. One school psychologist explained that she is usually the last one to evaluate the baby. "The team members who work at the facility during the day evaluate the baby at the same time; as a consultant I may do my assessment a week later. By that time the parents have already had to deal with the news.

"A lot of parents are very curious as to their child's test results. They ask, 'Can you tell me right now how my baby is functioning? Is my child really functioning at a three-month level?' Some parents are really anxious, and you have to be tactful.

"I feel most parents have already had the suspicion from the beginning. Hearing the news from a professional usually provides some sense of relief for the parents by confirming their suspicions."

Parents Seeking More than One Opinion: Families who are unhappy with a particular diagnosis should first discuss the issue with the professional(s) involved, then, if necessary, seek a second opinion from a qualified professional or from a diagnostic clinic.

A point made by Shore, Brice, and Love (1991) is that *parents, not tests, are the ultimate decision-makers about children.* "Parents certainly should be the final decision-makers," says a school psychologist. "But in reality the situation is very mixed. There are a few parents who are concerned and involved but ultimately differ with the decision made by the team."

Resistance may reveal itself in different forms. "One is a little bit of denial," explained one service provider. "It's very difficult to accept that you have a baby born with a handicapping condition who will never fit in with average children.

42 | A GUIDE TO MENTAL RETARDATION

"One family I worked with had a baby with Down syndrome. The baby wasn't diagnosed for several months, and once the baby was diagnosed, the parents had a hard time accepting the fact. Eventually they were able to accept the diagnosis to some degree, but later it was apparent that they still believed their baby was functioning like average children, even though the baby was delayed developmentally.

"Overall, however, I think long-term resistance is rare. Parents are generally looking for help and guidance however the team recommends. They are typically very receptive. They admit, 'I don't know how to do it.'

"The nice thing is that the team who works with the child ultimately works with the parents as well, working to educate them."

Are There Different Types of Mental Retardation?

Mental retardation is characterized by prolonged and severe deficits in thinking and reasoning (cognition), as well as deficits in meeting the needs of daily living (adaptive behavior). However, there are different levels of severity within mental retardation. When reading the characteristics that follow, it is important to remember that the mentally retarded are people first: they may have some things in common with others with mental retardation, but they also are individuals with unique histories, interests and skills, needs and desires.

A number of methods of classifying and identifying the levels of severity of mental retardation have been proposed over the past seventy-five years, and several different classification schemes are used today. The one most commonly used in the United States was developed by the American Association on Mental Retardation (AAMR).

The AAMR classification scheme has four levels of severity within mental retardation, each level based on a person's I.Q. score and adaptive behavior skills. These levels are mild, moderate, severe, and profound mental retardation.

Mild Mental Retardation: Mild mental retardation involves an I.Q. range of 55 to 69, associated with significant difficulties in adaptive behavior. About 75% to 85% of all people diagnosed as having mental retardation fall into this classification (Edgerton 1979).

People with mild mental retardation can usually speak and understand oral language, but they often have difficulty with more subtle use of language in terms of humor and sarcasm, relatively complex words and phrases, and the use of abstract concepts. Generally, people in this category can do very basic reading, writing, and arithmetic. Most people in this category require special education services in school. These training and educational programs need to be clear, concrete, and direct in order to be effective. Children and adults in this category are usually able to manage their own basic needs fairly well (for example, eating, dressing, personal hygiene, and basic communication).

In many ways, mild mental retardation is a handicapping condition most associated with school-age children. This level of retardation is most likely to be diagnosed when a child enters school. Researchers, such as anthropologist Robert Edgerton (1979), found that many people with mild retardation seem to fade into the general population after leaving school; they do not seem to request or need any kind of special services as adults.

Other adults with mild mental retardation, however, do need assistance with job training and support, housing, coping with the demands of daily living, and so on.

People with mild mental retardation often function relatively well as adults in society. Unfortunately, they are likely to have marginal employment and low income, thereby needing assistance coping with the demands of daily living. In many cases, this assistance is provided by friends, neighbors, relatives, coworkers, and others in the community. Robert Edgerton and other researchers discovered that this type of *informal assistance* is crucial for adults with mild mental retardation to survive in the community.

While adults with mental retardation make use of informal social support from other members of the community, these adults will frequently resent any attempt to label them or their children as mentally retarded or in need of special services. This is not surprising, given the expectation that adults in our society survive and take care of themselves and their families independently. The labels "retard" and "moron" typify abusive and denigrating language. Similarly, clinical, professional diagnoses such as mental retardation may create memories of rejection and humiliation for

44 | A GUIDE TO MENTAL RETARDATION

some. At times, these adults may respond positively to receiving assistance if the services are presented as services any adult in the community may need at one time or another.

Generally, adults with mild mental retardation find a niche for themselves in their communities. This does not mean their lives are free of problems. They are more likely to be unemployed or underemployed than others in the community, and they may not be able to cope with the inevitable stress and complication of daily living as well as other adults. This stress may become quite severe if the adult with mild retardation is a parent, especially if their own children have handicapping conditions or other difficulties.

Yet people with mild retardation may be able to cope well if they are able to develop an informal network of friends, neighbors, relatives, or others to provide help and support. Even with this support network, it is probable that adults with mental retardation living in the community will need some type of assistance during especially stressful times. These people may go for help to general community resources and agencies (for example, community social service offices, mental health centers, or the Salvation Army) rather than to agencies designed to provide services to people with mental retardation.

Moderate Mental Retardation: The other 20% to 25% of people diagnosed as having mental retardation fall into the categories of moderate, severe, or profound mental retardation. People with moderate mental retardation have I.Q. scores ranging from 40 to 54, and have even more significant deficits in the areas of adaptive behavior than people with mild retardation.

In general, people with moderate retardation are less able to use and understand oral and written language than persons with mild retardation. Individuals with moderate retardation may only be able to express themselves with a few words or short sentences. They may be able to read some signs or short sentences and recognize their written name, but their abilities in reading and arithmetic are likely to be very limited.

The person with moderate retardation usually needs help with more basic areas of adaptive behavior, such as personal hygiene, eating, and dressing. Most people with moderate retardation will need help and supervision during most of the day. One concern is that they may not be fully aware of commonplace dangers such as traffic or hot items on the stove.

Even with these difficulties and deficits, most people with moderate mental retardation enjoy socializing with friends, watching television, shopping, and going to the movies — many of the same activities enjoyed by other adults. They do not have to live in isolated places or large institutions, but can be happy, productive members of the community, living with their families, or in specialized apartments, group homes, and other small residences. While adults with moderate mental retardation may need continued training and support to help develop and maintain skills in adaptive behavior, they also can, with proper training and support, work and gain satisfaction from their work.

Severe Mental Retardation: Children and adults diagnosed as having severe mental retardation have I.Q. scores in the range of 25 to 39, and usually have significant difficulties with most areas of adaptive behavior. People in this category may be able to make their needs known with a very limited number of words or utterances, or through pointing or gestures. Many of those with severe retardation cannot speak at all.

Individuals with severe mental retardation generally need assistance with most of their daily needs, and have little understanding of commonplace dangers. Training and education for this population usually focus on developing skills so that the person can be as independent as possible in meeting his or her daily needs.

People with severe mental retardation, in spite of their limitations, also enjoy being part of their local communities. Residential programs, including specialized group homes and apartments, help those with severe retardation live in the community rather than in large institutions. Children with severe retardation can successfully live at home and attend special education classes in their local schools if the appropriate educational and family support programs are available.

Profound Mental Retardation: Individuals with I.Q.s of less than 25 are considered profoundly mentally retarded. They usually cannot speak; instead, they may make their needs known with very simple gestures and sounds.

46 | A GUIDE TO MENTAL RETARDATION

Individuals with profound retardation are often totally dependent on others to meet their needs. In general, they need round-the-clock care and support. Even with intensive training and assistance, most people with profound retardation will probably not become totally independent in *any* area of adaptive behavior.

It is important to recognize that, while people with profound retardation have many deficits and difficulties, they also enjoy the social contact of being in a community and being part of the activities of that community as much as possible.

Although the profoundly retarded have many complicated needs, there are specialized group homes and apartments which allow them to live in their local communities. Profoundly retarded children can live at home and be educated in special education programs in their local schools if the appropriate educational and family support programs are available. (For a good discussion of this issue, see Brown and Lehr 1989.)

Causation

People with mental retardation in the moderate to profound range — that is, those with I.Q.s of less than 55 and severe deficits in adaptive behavior — are more likely to suffer from an identifiable medical or genetic condition which caused or contributed to the condition. That majority (75% to 80%) of mentally retarded that can be classified as mildly retarded generally do not have an identifiable medical condition causing mental retardation.

Some recent research suggests, however, that there may be a genetic basis to almost 40% of mental retardation (Janicki 1988). As a result, the figures we will be quoting will probably change in the future as our understanding of mental retardation improves.

A Never-Ending Search: There are an enormous number of possible causes of mental retardation; in many cases, it is not possible to identify a single cause of the condition. Researchers have discovered, and continue to discover, many specific events, situations, and conditions which either cause mental retardation directly, or make it more likely that a particular individual will become mentally retarded.

(It is only possible to give a very brief overview of possible causes here, for the research is progressing so quickly in some areas that these discussions become somewhat outdated almost as soon as they appear in print. For a more comprehensive, and more technical, discussion, see Kavanagh 1988.)

The factors which cause or contribute to the development of mental retardation occur in three periods: before birth, during the birth process, and after birth. However, some factors may cause or contribute to the development of mental retardation both before and after the birth of a child.

Factors and Events Before Birth: Events and situations affecting the developing fetus fall into four main categories: (a) injuries and accidents; (b) genetic and metabolic factors; (c) exposure to toxic substances; and (d) exposure to infection.

(a) *Injuries and Accidents:* A significant injury or accident during pregnancy may put both the mother and the developing fetus at risk for significant medical problems, and long-term deficits and delays in both physical and mental development.

Malnutrition of both mother and fetus would be included in this broad category. It is clear that an inadequate diet during pregnancy may result in significant problems after birth, including mental retardation (Galler 1988). This problem is widespread in many Third World nations, but is also found in most of the developed nations, especially in the United States. Research has demonstrated that programs such as the Supplemental Food Program for Women, Infants, and Children (WIC) in the U.S., which help ensure that pregnant women have the proper diet and nutrition, not only reduce the incidence of mental retardation and other learning problems, but also are an extremely efficient use of taxpayer funds.

(b) *Genetic and Metabolic Factors:* There are hundreds of genetic conditions which may result in a child's mental retardation. Some of the more common genetic syndromes which can result in mental retardation include Down syndrome and Fragile-X syndrome. Another genetic condition is phenylketonuria (PKU), which involves the body's inability to properly metabolize certain amino acids. If untreated, PKU may result in severe mental retardation (Woo 1988). Less common metabolic conditions which may result in mental retardation include propionic acidemia, multiple carboxylase deficiency, and many others.

48 | A GUIDE TO MENTAL RETARDATION

A number of these conditions are treatable if diagnosed early enough. (For a brief but interesting discussion, see Nyhan 1988.) Some of these conditions can be diagnosed in the womb with the use of amniocentesis and other techniques.

(c) *Exposure to Toxic Substances:* If the mother and the developing fetus suffer exposure to toxic substances or environmental contaminants such as mercury, lead, some types of radiation, or many other industrial and agricultural chemicals, it can be a cause of mental retardation. Other types of exposure include substances such as alcohol, cocaine, narcotics, and certain types of prescription and nonprescription medications. Unfortunately, there seems to be an increasing number of infants and children who experience learning difficulties, including mental retardation, partially as a result of consumption of alcohol, narcotics, or certain medications during pregnancy.

Programs which reduce the risk of exposure to such contaminants as lead, as well as programs which help pregnant women get off, or stay off, alcohol and other drugs, are effective and reduce the costs associated with mental retardation.

(d) *Exposure to Infectious Agents in the Womb:* These infections may be viral, bacterial, or fungal, and could lead to serious handicaps later in life, or even death for the developing fetus.

Factors and Events During the Birth Process: These factors which may contribute to an individual's being diagnosed as mentally retarded later in life fall into three major categories: (a) exposure to infection; (b) injury during birth; and (c) premature birth and low birth weight.

(a) *Exposure to Infection:* It is possible for an infant to be exposed to infection during the process of childbirth. Such infections include viral diseases: for example, cytomegalovirus (CMV) and herpes simplex.

(b) *Injury During Birth:* There are a number of possible injuries an infant may suffer during the birth process, including oxygen to the brain being cut off because of the position of the umbilical cord.

(c) *Premature Birth and Low Birth Weight:* These usually occur simultaneously. Low birth weight infants are those who weigh less than 2,500 grams at birth and very low birth weight infants weigh less than 1,500 grams (a little over three pounds) at birth. Premature and low birth weight infants are at risk not only for mental retardation later in life but also for a number of serious, and in some cases life-threatening, medical conditions. A number of risk factors have been identified for mothers who are likely to have a premature and/or low birth weight infant. These factors include poverty and lack of prenatal care, use of alcohol and cigarettes during pregnancy, poor nutrition, and severe stress during pregnancy (Coates 1988).

This does not mean that all low birth weight or premature infants will develop mental retardation. Follow-up studies of even very low birth weight infants (Stahlman, Grogaard, Lindstrom, Haywood, and Culley 1988) found that the majority of these infants had normal intellectual development in later life. Still, there is a danger that infants in this category will develop mental retardation and other handicaps. Prenatal care for all pregnant women would not only reduce the number of individuals who develop mental retardation and other disabilities, but such prevention would be cost-effective as well.

Factors and Events During Childhood: Events and situations occurring after birth, and during the developmental stages of childhood, may also result in mental retardation. These events and factors include: (a) accidents and injuries; (b) exposure to environmental hazards and toxins; (c) malnutrition and other deprivation associated with poverty; and (d) illness and infection.

(a) *Accidents and Injuries:* Children can develop mental retardation as a result of automobile or pedestrian accidents, household accidents, near-drownings, and most tragic of all, some children develop mental retardation as a result of severe abuse and neglect.

(b) *Exposure to Environmental Hazards and Toxins:* Severe and prolonged exposure to lead, mercury, and other environmental hazards may contribute to the development of mental retardation and other handicapping conditions in certain cases.

(c) *Malnutrition and Other Deprivation Associated with Poverty:* Children who do not receive proper nutrition, or who experience a very deprived environment, also may develop mental retardation.

(d) *Illness and Infection* during childhood may result in mental retardation. Some adults also may develop conditions similar to mental retardation as a result of infection or illness. Technically,

50 | A GUIDE TO MENTAL RETARDATION

those who develop similar conditions during the adult years are not considered mentally retarded even though they may benefit from some of the services and training techniques used with adults with mental retardation.

Prevention

Research is continuing in many areas regarding the prevention of retardation and other disabilities, but we already have good research data on the effectiveness of many current prevention strategies. These include providing prenatal care to all pregnant women, accident prevention and safety programs; education and treatment programs designed to prevent and treat drug and alcohol dependency; reducing exposure to lead, mercury, and other toxins; and so on. Most of these prevention programs can be provided at a reasonable cost.

Mental retardation is best understood as a symptom of some type of damage to an individual's developmental process with no single cause, and there is generally no question of a cure. Yet although mental retardation is a lifelong disability, we must not forget that people with mental retardation are more *like* other people than they are different. Retarded children love to play with their friends, watch television, go to stores and to movies, just like other children. Retarded adults also like to be with their friends, go out and have a good time, earn their own money, and feel like a member of the community.

People with mental retardation, like people everywhere, are individuals with their own personal likes and dislikes, successes and failures. While these classifications of retardation are necessary to organize services and conduct research, these labels may become counterproductive, even destructive, if they imply that children and adults having mental retardation are so different that they have nothing in common with the rest of us.

Demographics

In the past, there has been a tendency — especially in some school programs — to diagnose mental retardation simply on the basis of the I.Q. score and not take into account the person's culture and adaptive behavior skills. At times this has resulted in a dispropor-tionate number of African-American, Native American, Hispanic, and lower-class children in general being diagnosed as mentally retarded and placed in special education classes.

This is not only a problem in the United States. In the United Kingdom, there has been controversy over the number of Irish and West Indian children diagnosed as mentally retarded in the public schools (Edgerton 1979), and similar situations have been reported in other countries. If there are a large number of false or inappropriate diagnoses of mental retardation, the estimates will be high and inaccurate.

Educated Estimates: A number of researchers estimated that about 3% of the general population is likely to be mentally retarded. Other researchers have criticized this figure, and estimate the true figure to be less than 2% of the general population. These esti-mates suggest that, while mental retardation is relatively common when compared to some other handicapping conditions, only a small proportion of the general population is likely to be mentally retarded in a given generation.

Mental retardation associated with a particular injury, illness, or genetic condition — which is likely to be moderate, severe, or profound mental retardation — seems to occur in *all* societies, so-cial, and cultural groups, and economic classes around the world.

While 75% to 80% of the mentally retarded population fall into the mild retardation category, it is believed that there was no clear physical, medical, or genetic cause for this type of retarda-tion. Recent research indicates that there may be more of a biolog-ical and medical basis to mild mental retardation than previously thought. (For a good discussion of this issue, see Bregman and Hodapp 1991.)

Poverty and Deprivation: In many cases, mild mental retardation seems most closely associated with poverty and deprivation. Ac-cording to Robert Edgerton: "It has been estimated that a child born in an impoverished rural area or in an urban ghetto is fifteen times more likely to be diagnosed as mentally retarded than a

52 | A GUIDE TO MENTAL RETARDATION

child from a middle-class suburban background" (1974, 4). We need to be careful here because poor children — especially those from ethnic or cultural minorities — may be inappropriately diagnosed as mentally retarded. But, even with this caution, most research appears to agree that mild retardation is associated with poverty.

In the poorest or most deprived area, only a relatively small proportion of the total population would be accurately diagnosed as mentally retarded. Research found that programs which reduce poverty and the many problems associated with poverty also have the benefit of reducing the most common type of mental retardation.

One psychologist who has worked with and written about the mentally retarded provides his own views on the issue of whether cultural deprivation is still a large factor of mental retardation today: "I have a bias on this issue. Years ago in a book I wrote, I talked about intelligence and that it isn't really normally distributed.

"Anyone with an intelligence below an I.Q. of 50 has some form of organic involvement. Autopsies of clients with I.Q.s below 50 have established brain injury in almost every single case. They truly are developmentally impaired.

"When discussing cultural problems, we're talking about people with actual I.Q.s above 50. We could go into a culturally disadvantaged home with a retarded child having an I.Q. of 35 — largely due to living in a one-room apartment; there's no stimulation for the child; none of the siblings are adequately cared for because both parents may have to work — but this child could attain an I.Q. of 50 with some work. I think it was one of those mythologies that cultural deprivation produces low I.Q.

"I worked at one residential home for twenty years, and we took the most disruptive, aggressive children from minority groups in New York City, and rarely was a child's I.Q. low; they were all about 70. And they came from the most horrendous conditions you'd ever want to see. If their I.Q. was really significantly below this, they truly were retarded *and* living in a disadvantaged home.

"There's always a case — some kid who was raised in a closet somewhere, who is tested and who can hardly speak. Then, with education, six months later he's starting to talk and come around. But those are rare exceptions. The average child — even growing up in a real impoverished environment — is fairly alert enough to do well on a number of subtests of some intelligence tests, such as the Weschler Intelligence Scale."

Gender: Another characteristic of mental retardation which seems to hold true around the world is that males are more likely to be mentally retarded than females. This higher ratio of males to females is also found in a number of other handicapping conditions in addition to mental retardation.

Acceptance

The general information we have provided so far illustrates some questions asked by parents which at the very least helps them move toward a point of acceptance. But the actual courses taken to reach this goal are as different and unique as the families who travel this road.

Some find acceptance and peace through active involvement in their child's training and education. Others find comfort in other family members, relatives, friends, and counselors. Still others form alliances with other parents in similar situations, sharing their strength and grief as they learn together. Regardless, when the support so desperately needed is discovered, the challenges of raising a mentally retarded child create great personal strength, courage, and wisdom, as their stories illustrate.

A Personal Story Revisited: Steven

Receiving Support: Just hours after Steven's birth, Mike and his wife, Julie, went for an evaluation by neonatologists. Their emotional devastation sent out a desperate signal for help. Fortunately for this couple the support was soon to come.

Mike recalls, "After we left, the medical center made an effort to be available. . . . We called a couple of times and asked them questions. They would call to check up with us as well.

54 | A GUIDE TO MENTAL RETARDATION

"Right away, following a suggestion by the medical center, we called the Down syndrome group. Within two weeks, on our own initiative, we had gone over and spoken to other parents.

"We had a lot of involvement from family, which is sort of both a blessing and a problem. It was a blessing because you really want to have support; you really want to have people acknowledge the birth and know that it is a time of problems. On the other hand, it takes a lot of energy to sustain talking with everyone, because everyone wants a piece of helping out — they want to know what is happening, they want to know about the baby. The amount of anguish that comes in just repeating things — keeping everyone informed — is a huge task. People don't want to wait and be on the sidelines; they want to find out what is happening. Their interest provides emotional comfort as well as takes mental energy."

Contact with Other Parents: "What we learned from other parents with babies with Down syndrome was that there were things we could do to help our son. We discovered that there is an early intervention program . . . which starts when the child is six-to-eight weeks old."

Seeking Answers: "We wanted to know what other people had experienced with their kids. We had a strong need to see other babies and older children with Down syndrome and to see what they were doing just to get ourselves through some uncertainties. We asked what parents were doing for their kids for intervention.

"Steven did not have the high medical needs common to most Down syndrome babies. The drama that surrounds some Down syndrome kids — especially where some may need open-heart surgery — was something we never had to deal with. In fact, Steven appeared to be a very healthy kid.

"I guess, in general, we wanted to know about other families with Down syndrome kids: Who are they? Where are they? With the information we obtained we were able to move towards getting Steven into an early intervention program."

A Personal Story Revisited: Mark

Recognizing the Needs of Other Parents: Mark's parents were able to place him in a special infant-stimulation program in their county. During this process, Al and his wife steadily became aware that they were not alone. Other parents were one step ahead of them, and still others were one step behind. Yet there appeared to be no organized system of help.

Al shared his story with us: "My wife and I were eating dinner one night, and I said to her, 'We've learned so much in the last three months about Down syndrome and the newborn. It took us dozens and dozens of phone calls and a lot of time trying to figure this stuff out. Wouldn't it be nice, if such a baby were born tomorrow, if those parents were able to call us? We could tell them in half an hour what it took us three months to learn.'

"We wondered how we could do this. The next time I was at the rehab center, I asked, 'Do you have any other parents here with babies with Down syndrome?' And, of course, they did. Then I said 'You know, we'd like to talk to them.' The staff was reluctant to give out names because of confidentiality. But this one therapist knew another couple who had made the same request."

Coming Together for Support: "She gave our names to them and their names to us. We talked, and found out their son was about six months older than ours. Then through work, we learned of another family with a boy who had Down syndrome, and we called them.

"One night, the six of us — three couples — got together and said, 'Between us, we know quite a bit about Down syndrome. It would be nice if we could share our experiences with a new family.'

"I called the hospital back, talked to the head nurse, asked her to have any new parents in a similar situation call us. One by one, just by word of mouth, we began to meet with other couples. By December, 1982, we had a meeting at someone's house with about five couples — each having children with Down syndrome — and we decided to form a parent group.

56 | A GUIDE TO MENTAL RETARDATION

"So then, through some agencies, we sent out an introductory letter. We picked a day and place to have a meeting in January and publicized it. Quite a few people showed up — I'd say between 40 and 45 people — a few professionals, but most of them parents of children with Down syndrome, some of the kids old, some still babies. We call ourselves the Down Syndrome Parent Group, but our meetings include anyone who is interested. We have parents of children with other disabilities because they don't have any other group to belong to and the problems are very similar. We became a tax-exempt, not-for-profit corporation."

Training in Parent Support: "Later we hired a social worker to train us. For example, we needed to learn to provide support to parents going through the grieving process — which is probably the first thing you do when you hear that your newborn is disabled. . . .

"Our group has become better at providing parent support. We contacted most of the hospitals in one county, and our group now covers three counties."

Breaking Down Barriers for Other Parents: "The activities of the group have changed as our kids have become older, since the most active people have been parents of kids roughly the same age. We couldn't get a lot of activity from parents of older kids; they already belonged to another group, and they didn't want to go to other meetings. Even though we've begged to become more involved with parents of older kids, it just hasn't happened.

"Those of us who started the group — some of our kids are now nine and thirteen — are focusing on educational issues at this point. Medical problems or dealing with infants aren't an issue anymore for the founding parents.

"We've had a lot of parents come into the group in the past two or three years with kids between infancy and three years old, and that's wonderful. These new parents are being trained to give support to newer parents. The founding members have been able to pass information and offer support while breaking the ice in the area of educational issues.

"It's amazing how, when a child reaches school age, you suddenly realize that a lot of your other concerns take the back burner. We had always wondered what things would be like for our son when he's twenty-two years old, but once he started school our thinking became more attuned to the here-and-now. He's five years old and having problems in school, so we're more focused on how he's going to make it through this particular school year."

The Parent Support Group

Developing Goals: "Our parent group decided when we drew up our constitutional charter that we would have five objectives: (1) To provide support to new parents; (2) To gather and disseminate information about Down syndrome and mental retardation; (3) To improve education for mentally retarded children; (4) To improve employment opportunities for people with mental retardation; and (5) To increase community awareness of mental retardation, specifically Down syndrome."

(1) *To Support New Parents:* "This goal was the one we accomplished first, and it is still our most active ongoing goal. We're going to have another training session with the social worker to train more parents to be support parents."

(2) *To Gather and Disseminate Information:* "We've been doing this for years, and we've been doing it very well. We received a grant a few years ago specifically to buy books, videotapes, and audiotapes, which we have available for lending. We have also bought books not for our library but to donate. We've donated several books to the library system and to high school libraries."

(3) *To Improve Education:* "This is an area where we've been very active for the last few years.

"We believe that segregating children with handicapping conditions is not the right thing to do. While it may be easier administratively, segregated education eliminates the possibility of social interaction with nondisabled children. To send our children away from their neighborhood schools, away from where their friends and siblings would be — to send them somewhere else just to be with other children like themselves is not in the best interest of the children."

(4) *To Improve Employment Opportunities:* "Most of the people who have been active in the group are those with younger

58 | A GUIDE TO MENTAL RETARDATION

children — although we have a few people with older children, though no one has gotten involved in addressing this goal yet.

"We do work with the local agencies, who have been doing a great job addressing the employment issue. Right now through supported employment with job coaches, one agency is finding jobs in real businesses instead of in the workshops for the retarded."

(5) *To Improve Community Awareness:* "We've formed a committee to develop a strategy for this goal. We've worked with the national group to have the month of October declared as National Down Syndrome Awareness month."

Educating Professionals: "A lot of pediatricians — a lot of doctors — will still tell the parent of a Down syndrome child that the best thing to do is not keep the baby, give it to the state, put it in an institution, put it up for adoption.

"Ten years ago, in Indiana, there was a girl born with Down syndrome and a closed esophagus. If she did not have surgery, a very simple procedure, she would die in a matter of days. For any normal child, the parents would want the surgery to be done. But in Baby Jane Doe's case the parents asked the doctor not to operate. Sure enough, ten days later the baby died. While not illegal, this was outrageous. Sadly enough, I know that the same thing happened again more recently. It illustrates that we still need to do a lot of education in the medical community."

"As more and more doctors have babies with Down syndrome, awareness of medical issues has increased. There are three or four physicians on the board of directors for the National Down Syndrome Congress who have children with Down syndrome. They're reaching out to the medical community, saying, 'Wait a minute, let's get rid of these old attitudes about Down syndrome. These children can lead a nice life. There's no reason not to give them all of the medical attention that any other child would get.'

"There are a lot of problems for kids with Down syndrome — heart defects, respiratory problems — and we try to collect information and get it into the hands of local doctors so that they are more aware of what to look for.

What Is Mental Retardation? | 59

"There are clinics that deal specifically with Down syndrome. So we tell our parents to take their baby to one of those clinics to have evaluations done by doctors who are familiar with Down syndrome. We give parents a list of medical issues that they can share with their pediatrician to make sure important characteristics are being evaluated."

Community Awareness and Job Opportunities: "I'm on the board of directors at a local rehabilitation program and we've talked to a lot of clients in the workshops who are not necessarily handicapped. If you ask them, 'Do you want to continue working in a workshop, or do you want to go out with a job coach and work at McDonald's or Burger King, or somewhere like that?' And every one of them would say they wanted to go to work out in the community."

"I know of cases where people have gone out into the community and worked; but after six months, they went back to the workshop. This happened not because they couldn't do the job, but because the people they were working with didn't really fully accept them.

"Let's say you're working at a fast food restaurant, and your coworkers who aren't handicapped don't respect you and don't help you and don't socialize with you. It would really be difficult working there. I could see where a handicapped person would say, 'Well, at least at the workshop I have friends to talk to.'

"That's why it is important for us to improve community awareness of disabilities."

Support for Mainstreaming: "People tend to be afraid of mentally ill or mentally retarded people. They don't want them living next door. I can show you newspaper articles of group homes almost near completion being burned down.

"We need to change this attitude. But I feel trying to change the attitude of adults is too large a task. I would rather devote my energy to raising a new generation of children who grow up with no prejudices. To do this we must begin in our schools.

"If you have children who have gone to school for twelve years, side-by-side with mentally retarded kids . . . physically handicapped kids . . . when those children grown up, they are not

60 | A GUIDE TO MENTAL RETARDATION

going to be prejudiced against mentally retarded adults. I feel a lot of acceptance in our younger generation already.

"Only then do I see us getting our handicapped people out into the community — not necessarily living in group homes, but living in apartments and with families.

"When I went to school I rarely saw a handicapped kid. I remember in high school seeing one of those yellow vans pulling up to the building and seeing half a dozen kids getting out of that van — they obviously were kids with mental retardation or some other disability. I remember seeing them going into a basement door and not seeing them again all day.

"When I think back now, I never really knew a handicapped kid when I was growing up. That's what we've got to change in the next generation. If kids go to school with handicapped kids from the time they are in kindergarten, just think what they are going to be like as adults. When they become employers they're not going to be afraid to hire someone who is handicapped." This will involve attitude changes on the part of millions of non-handicapped persons. I hope this book will inspire some of this change.

2

Infancy and Early Childhood

"The people who came to our home as part of the early intervention team gave us more hope than we could ever have imagined."

Having started life at a disadvantage, the child born with mental retardation requires assistance to develop certain skills necessary to function. This early intervention refers to educational and other services provided to young children (five years and younger) and their families. These programs are also designed to help families cope effectively with the demands of caring for a young child with a disability.

The federal government has been funding special education programs for young children since the middle of the 1960s. Many of these special education programs began as pilot projects in colleges and universities. Their success gave evidence that early intervention could be effective.

In 1975, Public Law (P.L.) 94–142 was passed by Congress. P.L. 94–142 mandated a free, appropriate public education for all students with handicaps who could not learn in regular classrooms. Although the provisions of P.L. 94–142 did not apply to children younger than age six, the legislation included incentive grants for states to develop educational programs for infants and toddlers with handicaps.

62 | A GUIDE TO MENTAL RETARDATION

With the passage of the Education of the Handicapped Act Amendment of 1986 (also known as P.L. 99–457), states were required to develop programs to serve three- to five-year-old children, and eventually to serve infants and toddlers with handicaps from birth to age three. The cost of these services was to be shared by the federal and state governments and, in some cases, also by the county and municipal governments.

The number of early intervention services vary from state to state since some states had fairly comprehensive services even before the passage of P.L. 99–457. Which agency actually provides the services will also vary greatly. In some states, one state agency provides or coordinates all early intervention services from birth to age five. Other states have one agency providing services from birth to three, and another agency providing early intervention for ages three to five. In many states and regions, the government does not directly administer the early intervention programs, but contracts with various nonprofit groups to provide these services in a particular area or region.

The Role of the Federal Government

The federal government has been very helpful in encouraging and supporting the development of early intervention services. But there is a danger that families and other advocates will assume that the federal government will carry all the responsibility in their county or state. Even though there are federal requirements and mandates, the early intervention programs will need the support of parents as well as advocates in state and local legislatures.

Hebbeler, Smith, and Black (1991), in their summary of federal policies regarding early intervention, illustrate the situation well: "Federal policy can point the way and certainly can help with funding, but the commitment that ultimately will achieve the final goal must come at the state and local levels" (p. 111).

Special education programs are designed primarily to provide educational services to infants, toddlers, young children, and their families. P.L. 99–457 mandates that certain support services, such as physical or occupational therapy, speech and language therapy, transportation, and other services, be provided if these services help attain an educational goal.

Infancy and Early Childhood | 63

In general, the early intervention programs are available to those children who need comprehensive educational services. Parents in doubt should check with their local agency responsible for early intervention services since policies and services will vary from state to state and region to region within a state. If you do not know which agency provides early intervention services, the local school district, or a United Way office, should be able to provide this information.

A Closer Look

The following information is based on the comments of a psychologist and writer, and an interview with the director of Education Services at an ARC Center and a coordinator of Early Intervention Services at an ARC Center.

Q: What is your background?

"I'm a Special Educator. I started work at the early intervention program about eight years ago. The program has grown to such an extent that it required more teachers, more therapists, and someone to coordinate all the services that are provided to our program. And so I've moved from being a Special Education Teacher in an early intervention program to coordinator of those services."

"My certification is in Special Education. I then went on to get a certificate as a school district administrator."

Q: What constitutes effective early intervention?

"Early intervention is not the same as assisting the handicapped child to function more normally. Early intervention assists the *family* to function more normally. If a husband and wife didn't have access to all the services that now exist for their retarded child, they'd have to do all the work themselves; this would put undo stress on their relationship and on their family unit."

64 | A GUIDE TO MENTAL RETARDATION

Q: What age group does the ARC Center serve?

"The ARC Center serves children from birth to twenty-one years of age. Early Intervention Services has a home-based program that serves children from birth to three years of age. The Center-Based Preschool Program serves children from under two years of age up until five years of age. A center-based program is a truly education model: a child is placed in a classroom setting with a special education teacher, a teacher assistant, and teacher-aids. The number of staff per classroom depends upon the number of children in the classroom.

"The children are also eligible to receive related services, such as physical therapy, occupational therapy, and speech therapy. We also provide music therapy and some adaptive physical education. We have several children here who require services of a vision specialist as well."

Q: What populations do you reach, and how are parents informed of your services?

"Our outreach has not been very good. That is something we are trying to improve.

"A lot of children are referred here by the New York State program called Early Childhood Direction Centers, which is funded under the State Education Department. Their primary role is to match parents of children with appropriate services. This is probably the largest source of our referrals.

"We occasionally get referrals through the public health department. Sometimes we do get referrals directly from a physician. Sometimes we get a call from a parent or family member who has a question or concern about the development of his or her child. Occasionally we get a call from the Department of Social Services.

"The population we've seen an increase in recently is parents with developmental disabilities who have children at risk for developing those kinds of disabilities. We've seen an increase in the number of those kinds of 'borderline' kids."

"We've been finding a lot of referrals from rehabilitation programs for parents involved with substance abuse, and we have been doing screenings and evaluations for children of parents in these programs."

Infancy and Early Childhood | 65

"This is a new population for us." And, of course, every population has its own particular problem.

Q: Who pays for these services?

"In New York State, we are funded through family court in the county where the parents reside. The family actually has to petition family court for services for their child under the age of three.

"This petition needs to be signed by a physician and a psychologist, stating that the child falls into one of the eleven categories of need that the Department of Education says qualifies as a handicapping condition. The child, if he meets at least one of these handicapping conditions, is then eligible to receive services. The tuition for each child is paid by the county, and the county is reimbursed 50% by the state.

"Federal legislation from several years ago (P.L. 99–457) requested all states to adopt a different kind of system. New York has been slow in following suit, except for children age three to five. New York put jurisdiction for those students in the school district where the child resides, under a Committee on Preschool Special Education. But still, the school district has no financial responsibility for those kids; they have the task of approving placement for them.

"There is no cost to families themselves for any services in this type of program *at this time.* There is legislation pushing for families to *have* to pay into that, but there is major controversy around the issue."

Q: For children ages three and under, what is the new system which inevitably will replace the current system of funding?

"New York State has a bill right now that gives the State Health Department the responsibility to set up the new programs for birth to age three.

"Most of the programs now providing services to those kids are educational programs, such as ours, and have always worked under the State Department of Education. The orientation of the

66 | A GUIDE TO MENTAL RETARDATION

Health Department is going to be much more of a medical model, as opposed to an educational model.

There have been counterproposals from some groups. . . . These groups want the system to build on existing models, rather than trying to re-create the wheel by falling back on the medical model. The kinds of issues that we face with these kids aren't always seen by people in the medical profession; they have such an orientation to fixing things. We're concerned that kids aren't going to be able to get the services they really need.

"One problem with the model as it exists now through family court is that there is no consistency from one county to another. It is very hard to assure that all the children will be able to locate services on an equal basis. On this level, it is good to see new legislation where all children throughout the state would get equal access. But it won't help to do away with services that already exist, or to implement fee-for-service where parents have financial responsibility. One of the things they are saying is that parents would need to use insurance to pay for these services."

"A recent conference looked at the difference between services being provided for children ages birth to three and the new proposed legislation. They described a shift from *child-centered* programming to *family-focused* programming. The move is toward seeing the child as part of a family and working with the family as a whole — all of their needs and all of their strengths — as opposed to just coming in to do therapy with the child."

Family-focused therapy is training a parent to work with their child. Our family-directed therapy, on the other hand, involves going into the home and providing the family with all the necessary information which, ultimately, will help the *family* make all the decisions and choices.

One of the big goals in services for handicapped children is to create the *least restrictive environment.*

There is concern over *integration* and *inclusion*, and what constitutes integration and inclusion for a child under age three.

"We went to a conference . . . where there were people talking on both sides of this Early Care vs. Early Start proposal now being sponsored. . . . People started talking about inclusion for kids under age three."

For center-based programs there may be the concern about transportation to the site. Fortunately, in most cases parents are eligible for transportation services. But if a child is physically so fragile that he or she may not be able to be taken out of the home, then the child would best be served by home-based programs.

Q: What situations are you finding in the public school systems with the kids who are coming from early intervention programs?

"It depends upon the population. Over the last few years, the preschool children that we've been serving have tended to be more mildly retarded. Those kids will definitely leave here, once they've reached school age, and go into public school classes. Ninety-nine percent of these children will always require special education services of some kind.

"The kids who will stay here are becoming fewer and fewer. They tend to be the most severely, multiply handicapped children — many very physically impaired, some with behavioral issues or severe retardation.

"The number of school-aged kids that we serve is going to continue to dwindle because the programs for school-age are beginning to provide services. Over time, we will become a preschool program because of the mandates that the schools serve school-age kids.

"When children turn preschool age — if they have been with us prior to age three in the family court-funded program — the process is that the family, in theory, contacts the school district to let them know that there is a preschool-age child who requires services. We forward evaluations to them.

"The general rule is that the child who has already been with us would probably stay with us for preschool services. It doesn't have to be that way, however; the parent has the option of choosing any preschool program that is approved to provide services for that child (in terms of the child's handicapping condition) and which feels that it could most appropriately meet that child's needs.

"When the child is turning school age, it then becomes the responsibility of the school district to actually do the evaluation. It's their responsibility to determine whether they have a program that is appropriate for that child within their district. If not, they need to find what other services are available for that individual, and then they have to contract for the provision of those services."

68 | A GUIDE TO MENTAL RETARDATION

Q: What are some of the joys and frustrations of an early intervention program for parents and teachers?

"Not enough is a good answer to this question: Not enough time; not enough resources; not enough money. The lack of resources includes human resources as well as financial. There's not enough time, in that it is so easy to get caught up in the routine of what you have to do. For example, our program requires each teacher to make two home visits a week, but you don't have the time to be creative and come up with new approaches."

"I see the frustrations of not enough, as well, but it also is because the field is still so new. There's a lot of freedom to explore and be creative in it. That's what is really exciting from all perspectives: parents, children, and staff. There's a lot going on — a lot of shifting and moving. It is so *not static* that it is really exciting to be in this field right now.

"Things should always be shifting and changing in this field, and there should be a whole continuum of options. There shouldn't be only one way to help this population. That's why legislation can be scary; if it really fixes things, interventions may become stale."

"Our program, realistically speaking, is fixed to a large extent. Our home-based model follows [regulations], but some more flexibility would be nice.

"We've just released some kids with the county who had cognitive needs on target, which was exciting — we feel good about what our program has done for them. But now, all of a sudden, their eligibility for services becomes questionable, even though their motor needs may be significantly impaired. In order for a child to qualify for this kind of program, in theory, they are supposed to be functioning lower than their chronological age.

"It would be nice, even if your area of need is only in the motor area, if you could still qualify for special services. But the typical response is if a child doesn't need an educationally modeled program, send him or her for out-patient physical therapy."

Q: What are parents' and families' common questions about early intervention programs and services?

Infancy and Early Childhood | 69

"Parents ask us, 'What are you going to do for my child? What do I need to do? How are your going to help me to do this? What are the benefits to my child? Is this going to cost me any money?'

"Often parents will ask 'Who will my child be down the road?' One of the first things any team member going into that home tries to do is bring the parent to the present, to deal with the child's needs at the present moment, instead of thinking or worrying about later on. There's plenty of time to do that."

"If you have a kid with a disability, it is absolutely one of the most traumatic experiences that you'll ever have in your life. And if you can handle that, the rest is easy. I think it gives you a different perspective on everything.

"The parent of a child recently diagnosed raising these sorts of issues about their child's development is understandably going through a very tough time. People working in close relationship such as teachers and therapists have to be more than teachers and therapists. They have to be equipped to be counselors."

"Most of the families I work with — just about all of them — upon meeting them, have said, 'I've never been with or around or known an infant with a handicap until my own was born.' From the beginning what you're doing is introducing them to information about handicapping conditions in general, about the specific handicapping condition their child has, informing them about the different therapies available with which they will be involved. In general, we try to make parents aware of the terminology and explain what the services really are, as well as be a resource for information.

"While most parents do ask many questions about the future, many discover it really isn't what they need to focus on. At the time, however, it's the stage they're working through. We try to help them keep coming back to what's happening now. Sometimes *they* don't even realize what their needs are, what their assets are, or the importance of their assets.

"Another important issue in working with parents is connecting parents with other parents for support, information, and empowerment. I think one of the most important parts of an early intervention program is getting parents to meet with one other parent, several other parents, a group of parents — it doesn't matter how many. It doesn't even matter if there are similarities in

70 | A GUIDE TO MENTAL RETARDATION

their children's handicapping conditions, just someone who understands. It doesn't matter what a professional knows, or how much they've studied, or how much they've working with families of handicapped children, experiencing it firsthand provides something qualitatively different and beneficial. That really is an important issue, especially early on."

"We've also noticed that parents who, early on, have been participants in an early intervention program become much more vocal, much more actively involved in their children's educational process after they've transitioned out of an early intervention program into school age. We've got a whole new group of parents here who are very vocal and very active in their children's education.

"It really helps to have parents see the importance of themselves and the whole family in all this. We come in to work *with* them, not to tell them what to do. This is a very important point."

"We try not to see early intervention as something apart from their daily lives, but something that is integrated *into* it. These are parents raising children just like anyone else: You have a teenager, you integrate the insanity of life with a teenager; you have a child with special needs, you integrate that reality and the requirements it brings with it."

"Also, we try to support that kind of situation where a parent reaches a point where they say, 'I can't do this anymore.' We do whatever we can to come up with resources."

"It's each to their own possibilities and limitations. It's not like we try to make them all ideal parents of special-needs children.

"One important thing is for the professionals to give more credence to parents and their observations, their feelings, their knowledge, their information. I think, over the years, it has been the professional coming in and being *the one who knows*. Now I think the tables are turning — slowly. Parents are the ones who really live with these children, and these are the people who know far better than we do. And being the parent is *much* harder than being the professional."

"While there are two extremes — passive to militant — there are those parents who are inquisitive enough to ask what their options are, then ask for help in selecting the best of what is available

Infancy and Early Childhood | 71

of how to make it even more available. Some parents are willing to put a good amount of effort into it to change things."

"It is important that parents know that they need not hesitate to advocate for themselves or their children when there is a concern. They need not be afraid to confront the professional even when the professional is saying, for example, that nothing is wrong.

"Gut instinct, more often than not, is going to be correct. If the parents really feel that something is awry, they might want to keep looking until they find that person who can help — and it won't necessarily be a doctor."

"In dealing with the youngest population in early intervention, it's important to use a team approach. We're moving from what we call *interdisciplinary* to *multidisciplinary* teams, and finally to *transdisciplinary* treatment teams — which at this point is considered the best you can achieve — with people really working with, engaging, consulting, learning, even training one another about their discipline. A family receiving services could get a very well-rounded approach.

"When [one] state followed the federal mandate to provide services for birth to three, the Health Department set up what they called regional planning groups. It was divided into geographic areas. It was a great idea, a lot of discussion went on, and one of the things they came up with was a subcommittee called Personnel Training.

"We realized that our ability to provide services was significantly limited when everyone is trained only in their particular field. We felt that all the different disciplines really needed to learn as much as they could about each other: for example, special education teachers working with very young children needed to learn a lot about motor development.

"When working with very young handicapped children, you need a lot of medical background. Occupational therapists and physical therapists get a lot of medical background, but speech therapists are only trained in oral motor issues. Special education teachers don't always get all the medical background they need either. And everyone can benefit from some social work training.

"It can also become confusing to the family. They may think, 'When I diaper the baby, I should do it this way. And when I feed the baby, I should do it that way,' instead of all of us working

72 | A GUIDE TO MENTAL RETARDATION

together on *all* the different skills in the daily routine of the child. We could all be contributing, as opposed to the physical therapist saying 'do it this way,' and the occupational therapist saying 'do it that way.'

"If a child has special needs in language skills, and since the teacher is the person in direct contact with that child, it doesn't make sense to wait for that once-a-month visit from the speech therapist to provide the kind of training the child and parent need. Ideally, the speech therapist could come in and train everyone working with the child about things that we could be doing."

"We tend to consider the teacher to be the generalist. She is able to draw more from all the disciplines because they all constitute education for that kid. You can't take out the motor part; you can't take out the cognitive part; you can't take out the speech and language part. You can't treat them all separately. They *are* the education for that child. So, the teacher — whether by training or by personality — accepts that role as being the generalist, and he or she tries to get all the disciplines to work together on a regular basis, to get all the information needed, and make sure that the disciplines are generalizing to each other. From our model program, the teacher has the most important role."

"A perfect example is working with the child with feeding problems. Parents will think you're just working on feeding issues with the child. But you're also working on eye contact; you're working on social skills — interaction between parent and child; you're working on the posture of the child; you're working on the fine-motor skills of the child; you're working on getting the child to respond in a particular way to indicate what he or she wants. Many different areas are being addressed within that one task. And showing this to a parent — just the feeding alone — allows them to see how all the different skills can be worked on at once."

"An important message that we've tried to get across to families — but isn't often heard — is that *more* doesn't always mean *better* when it comes to services. Particularly with the shortage of some services, such as speech therapy. Our approach is that a teacher should be a generalist; teachers can conduct a lot of these services to some extent.

"However, parents seem to be saying: 'I want my kid to get eight hours of speech therapy, seven days a week.' Often we have

Infancy and Early Childhood | 73

to say, 'Yeah, we'd like to give you more, but we can't. But that doesn't mean your child is losing — more doesn't have to mean better.' It's a real hard point to drive home to parents.

"They put too much trust in the professionals to fix everything. They have to realize the importance of what *they* are doing on a regular basis, and that their efforts can come to the same ends. Whether the parent is the one trying to get the child to imitate sounds, or the speech therapist is the one trying to get the child to imitate sounds — it's the same thing. Just because the therapist is doing it doesn't mean it's better."

Early Intervention: A Parent's Perspective

Mike, who talked about his experiences as a new parent, describes his family's involvement in different services provided through early intervention programs.

"Our first efforts at early intervention involved a physical therapist who came to our home twice a week for one hour each sitting. Down syndrome babies, due to their low muscle-tone, have an inability to make certain movements; they don't move through the stages easily. Therefore, the physical therapist, for the majority of the time, would work with the baby with us at her side as she was getting him to use some of his muscles.

"The early intervention program was center-based and was later expanded to include at-home intervention. They also have a toddler program and a three-year-old program, so that you can continue with that intervention process as your child grows older.

"We used our insurance to have a speech therapist begin work with Steven when he was one-and-a-half years old. Basically, this was a language stimulation program, done in our home, until Steven was about five years old. We had more control over this; we had the opportunity to find the therapist that we wanted rather than use whoever was available — not that we didn't have a good experience with the therapist at the early intervention program.

"Steven was also involved with a preschool language stimulation program at age three. . . .

"Generally speaking, it has been our attempt to have Steven with kids who are good models for him — kids he can learn from — as well as having good teachers. That program met that goal for us.

74 | A GUIDE TO MENTAL RETARDATION

"We are still concerned that things could blow up in our faces. But in some ways that is a concern with self-contained classrooms too: that things will fall apart because there are a lot of high-need kids who are very demanding on the teacher. My child may have a very bad year because of a stage he's going through.

"In some sense, our anxiety level during the years when he was less included was as high — or higher — than it is now. The educational program for handicapped children is very different at some schools now than it was five years ago. It is not clear how the system will change year after year.

"It's being designed as we go: By the school. By us. By the school and us together. By the teachers. By the speech therapist in the school. . . . It's a big discovery process."

A Child's First Experience with Inclusion

Mike continues, "At four years old, Steven went to his second year of preschool for half a day. For the other half of the day, he was in a Head Start classroom with seventeen other kids as part of an inclusion program. It was his first major experience being with 'normal' kids. With his handicap, Steven required extra planning and, at times, extra staffing by the Head Start program.

"Steven's adjustment went well. He had a particularly short attention span; he was obstinate; and his speech was less understandable. He was not yet toilet trained, and they had to deal with that.

"Steven didn't appear to notice that he was any different from the kids around him. He doesn't make that observation now either; he does not say, 'Why are they doing that while I'm doing this?' except in the framework of, 'I would like to do that.' [Feeling different] is not something that has been part of Steven's self-observation. He's working in a more concrete world than the other kids. Feeling different is not an emotional event that he has had to deal with.

"The other kids wouldn't make that generalization about themselves either. Three- and four-year-olds are not that self-observant nor are they concerned with other kid's behaviors. What they will do is react to someone picking on them. They don't go home and say, 'Hey, there's a boy in my class who doesn't speak very well.'

Infancy and Early Childhood | 75

"One of Steven's strengths is that he has a wonderful smile. And he is very exuberant. Because of this, he creates a lot of positive attention for himself from other kids and other adults. They like to be around someone who is smiling."

Head Start

Another avenue taken years back to provide a service for children who are behind — whether due to mental retardation or cultural poverty — is the Head Start program. The following is based on a conversation with the former assistant director of an early childhood program.

Q: What were the responsibilities of your position?

"As the administrator, my responsibility was directing five Head Start centers, each of which included a day-care center component.

"As director of those programs I was responsible for the supervisor of each center. Prior to this, my experience as a teacher of very young kids — ages three to six — was something that prepared me to administer programs that served those children."

Q: Who was served by the programs you administered?

"To receive funding for the Head Start centers, we were required to provide services to low-income eligible children and children, regardless of their income, who had a diagnosed handicapping condition. The classrooms were composed of these two groups.

"Both groups were together. There was no differentiation in terms of the schedule or groupings of kids. Some tasks were handled differently, depending upon each child's needs."

Q: How did Head Start begin? What is its focus?

"The Head Start movement began in 1965 as part of President Johnson's 'War on Poverty.' At this time, schools were still putting handicapped kids into self-contained classrooms when these kids reached public school age.

76 | A GUIDE TO MENTAL RETARDATION

"The program with which I was involved was really doing a lot of work trying to include children with handicapping conditions long before the schools were attempting to do this. The children who left Head Start went on to public school, usually into kindergarten. Head Start, for the most part, operated separately from the public school system.

"The focus of Head Start is to involve parents in as many ways as possible with their child, and to provide services to families in need. This will include social service referrals, nutritional information and assistance, and assistance with problem-solving and parenting skills, to name a few.

"The Head Start program is funded and staffed to help multi-need families who are income eligible. In addition, it provides extra support for families who aren't necessarily high-need families but who are still low-income."

Q: What is the status of Head Start today?

"Head Start continues to get a lot of positive publicity nationally. It is getting increased funding, and it is one of the few points that President Bush will fund that are part of the 'War on Poverty' program.

"Most of the programs that were started have been eliminated or have been reduced so much that they really aren't important in this country's efforts to help families that are low-income anymore.

"Because the money actually comes from the federal government to the state government and finally to the local agencies, some states have started pre-kindergarten programs for four-year-olds, which is similar to Head Start in some ways, and reaches additional kids. New York State is part of this."

Q: Has Head Start prevented further cases of mental retardation caused by cultural deprivation?

"Today, the medical basis for mental retardation is certainly evident for kids who have Down syndrome and for other sources of retardation. Kids can develop retardation because of medical sit-

Infancy and Early Childhood | 77

uations in early childhood, or prenatal conditions, which may have some environmental causes.

"These days, people are classified as retarded according to their ability to learn. But I'm not sure Head Start changes the *ability* to learn. It may intervene with that child earlier to help them have more years of learning and have a more positive experience."

Parenting a Mentally Retarded Child: The Emotional Aspects

For most parents, the day they learn the diagnosis of mental retardation for their infant or toddler is probably one of the most devastating days of their lives. Parents have reported having a number of intense feelings and concerns when they were told their child was mentally retarded — grief, denial, anger, anxiety, shame, loneliness, a need to blame someone or something, as well as other feelings unique to each parent and family.

Researchers and clinicians have proposed a number of different stages in how families adapt to the diagnosis of mental retardation for their child. Some have proposed three stages of adjustment; others have proposed up to seven.

One clinician maintains that family members experience sorrow and grief throughout the life cycle of the child, while others reject this concept and argue that most families move beyond sorrow and grief to constructive action.

Other professionals find little evidence to support any of these theories or stages of adjustment; they argue that theories are of little use in constructively working with families. (For a good discussion of this issue, see Turnbull and Turnbull 1990, 108–110.)

There is helpful information from research on families. We know that, if a child is diagnosed very young, the grief reactions seem to be more intense. But if the child is diagnosed as a toddler, or in kindergarten or school, the parents, while still experiencing some grief, are more likely to experience some relief at the confirmation of a diagnosis they may have suspected for some time (Turnbull and Turnbull 1990).

We also know that parents and families are unique and that we simply cannot apply theories or offer help without getting to know the special situation of each family. There is also evidence that families naturally want empathy and understanding when they hear the diagnosis for the first time, but that they also want an honest and open discussion of the diagnosis. Attempts to "shield" the family from the diagnosis seem to make the situation worse.

Professionals need to consider balance: "The professional needs to balance hope with realism, which is a very difficult thing to do when you're dealing with young parents. You don't want them to give up all hope, because then they won't bond with their infant. On the other hand, you don't want the parents to have unrealistic hopes. You need to walk the fine line of giving hope but not unrealistic hope," said one psychologist.

"Sadly, a lot of professionals are not trained to do this. Most of the time, the first person who deals with the infant is a pediatrician, whose whole focus is normal development. When he or she sees a child that is abnormal, there's a certain level of identification for that pediatrician with the parent. It's like his or her child too. Often the pediatrician plays down the child's handicap and goes too far in the direction of giving the parents unrealistic hope."

The evidence indicates that families who receive information about their child's diagnosis in an honest and sympathetic way make a quicker and healthier adjustment to dealing with the diagnosis (Turnbull and Turnbull 1990, 109).

Learning to Cope: A Process

While each family and family situation is unique, there are ways for parents to help themselves and others cope with the diagnosis of mental retardation in an infant or young child. This involves a process of obtaining and confirming information on the diagnosis; identifying, labeling, and sharing feelings; finding strength; keeping perspective; and working together.

These events do not necessarily move through a specific sequence. Parents and family members may or may not move through the process of learning to cope in a similar fashion. Once certain parts of the cycle are completed, they may or may not need to be addressed again.

The issue of confirming the diagnosis and obtaining accurate information, for example, may be resolved for a time, but can emerge again as an issue for the family, perhaps years later. Also, family members will probably be involved in different parts of the coping cycle concurrently. This does not mean that the family members are failing to cope, nor does it mean they are not going through the coping process as a family unit.

Confirming the Diagnosis

The first part of the coping process is obtaining and confirming information about the diagnosis. Some families receive an honest, sensitive, and accurate diagnosis and assessment of the needs of their child. Others may spend years trying to obtain information. Parents should be very cautious of a diagnosis that seems too quick, too vague, or doesn't make sense.

Unfortunately, there still are situations where some professionals make snap diagnoses with little information. If a professional makes a diagnosis of mental retardation based on a quick physical examination — or even worse, simply by looking at the child — there is good reason to doubt that professional's competence and understanding of mental retardation.

A quick diagnosis is not *always* inaccurate, but does indicate the need for a second opinion. If the professional will not take the time to discuss the diagnosis, and the possible implications of the diagnosis for you and your family, you should also be concerned, and seriously consider getting a second opinion.

If you have a strong feeling that the diagnosis is based on limited or wrong information, it is important to seek a second opinion. Your original feeling may or may not be correct, but parents should learn to trust their instincts and obtain more information or a second opinion when they have doubts.

Seeking a second opinion does not necessarily mean that you believe the professional making the original diagnosis was wrong or incompetent. In my experience, professionals who are secure in their knowledge and skill often will encourage families to obtain a second opinion.

Some professionals, in an attempt to "spare" the parents, will use vague or general terms when they really want to diagnose mental retardation. They might make very general statements such as "everything will be okay," or "the child will grow out of it,"

80 | A GUIDE TO MENTAL RETARDATION

even when they have a strong suspicion that mental retardation is the most accurate diagnosis.

The research available suggests that parents are better able to deal with an honest diagnosis even when it is wrong than with an attempt to hide reality. Even when faced with dishonest reassurances, most parents know when there is really something wrong with their child. Dishonest reassurances can cause parents to lose confidence in all professionals.

Parents should be cautious if the professional is too quick to reassure them. Sometimes, professionals cope with their own anxieties and insecurities about a diagnosis of mental retardation by passing off the diagnosis as "no big deal," or by promising that "all kinds of services are available."

One program director explains: "The biggest problem with having a handicapped child is that your expectations are that whatever disorder he has will respond to the various habilitation efforts you expose the child to.

"If professionals hold out unrealistic hopes for the child, they can often precipitate depression. As the child gets older and the mother and father see that their child isn't attaining a normal level of functioning, they may feel guilt that they didn't go to the right treatment center, or guilt that they didn't put enough effort into the program. . . .

"Anyone looking at literature over the ages can see what have been reported as 'miracle cures' in the area of mental retardation. There was a time when it was thought that certain vitamins would help the retarded. . . .

"There has always been — and always will be — some scientist who wants to make a name for himself by coming out with some kind of miracle cure."

The hard truth is that mental retardation is a disabling, life-long, handicapping condition; it is indeed a "very big deal" for the person and his or her family.

Services may be available in the local community, or the promise of these services may come from a dimly remembered book or pamphlet, from a public service announcement, or from information about another community or state. If parents are offered services by a professional, they should press for details and specifics. If there are no convincing details forthcoming, or the topic is dropped abruptly, the promise of services is probably based on the professional dealing with his or her own anxieties rather than a real knowledge of the service system.

At the same time, there may be appropriate services in the local community, and parents should contact local agencies for information (several national resources are listed on pages 251–254).

The other side of meaningless reassurance is the equally destructive, overly pessimistic approach. Professionals who are too pessimistic may be correct in the diagnosis of mental retardation, but give families an unduly bleak perception of the life a person with mental retardation can lead.

These professionals may have good intentions, but their knowledge of mental retardation is usually limited or seriously out of date. One sign of a potential problem in this area is if the professional tries to predict how an infant or preschool child with mental retardation will function as an adolescent or adult. The more specific this prediction is, the more likely it is that the professional may not have a lot of current accurate information about mental retardation.

Such a list as this of potential problems and mistakes of professionals may seem to imply that the professionals involved in these situations are incompetent or ignorant, but in most cases this is not true. Professionals who make these mistakes are usually motivated by a genuine concern for the child and his or her parents and are trying to make a difficult situation as easy as possible for everyone involved.

There are also many cases where professionals try to give families as much accurate information as possible, only to find the information rejected.

Professionals, like everyone else, can make mistakes. Families should not have unrealistic expectations of what professionals can do, or what information they can provide, but should accept that professionals do not have all the answers.

Identifying and Sharing Feelings

Parents of a young child with mental retardation are under enormous stress, especially around the time of the diagnosis. It is understandable that many parents want to draw back into them-

82 | A GUIDE TO MENTAL RETARDATION

selves, unable — or unwilling — to share their feelings of grief and pain with their family, relatives, or friends. This withdrawal may be a necessary part of the adjustment process.

This withdrawal if it lasts too long can cut the family off from many potential sources of help and encouragement. The most destructive form of withdrawal is when one parent shuts him or herself off from the other in an attempt to cope with the situation.

A parent may express tremendous anger at the real or imagined failures of a spouse or professional, whom he or she blames for the mental retardation. Some parents will express anger or shame about the child with mental retardation.

There are many different ways of identifying, labeling, and sharing feelings. Certainly not all parents are comfortable with professional counselors or even parent support groups. But friends, family members, trusted neighbors, members of the clergy, and others may be able to help with this process of coping with feelings.

Sharing feelings is an important first step in the process of coping for most parents. There are parents who may never be ready to share these feelings, and this sharing should never be pressured, coerced, or used as a condition for the parent or child receiving services.

There is also the danger that the sharing of feelings is seen as a solution and as an end in itself. The sharing and labeling of feelings should be the springboard for constructive action for the parents.

"I was constantly amazed by the attitude of some professionals and students from various human service disciplines who asked about the services we provided," said a coordinator of a family services program. "These professionals and students had no concept that parents of children and adults with mental retardation would need, or want, services beyond the opportunity to express feelings in a support group.

"In response, I told them that relatively few parents were interested in support groups focused on the expression of feelings. This is not to imply that support groups should not be available to those who want them; however, parents usually find a way of labeling and expressing feelings without the help of counselors or groups.

Infancy and Early Childhood | 83

"Expression of feelings is an important part of the coping process for most parents, but this should not be seen as an end in itself."

For example, infants with mental retardation may not bond as quickly with their mothers, and may find it hard to attain independence. "The retarded child often has difficulty bonding because he doesn't have the complete sensory apparatus that the normal infant has to bond. He may not be able to fixate in the gazing phase of attachment. He may not be able to play the kinds of hand-regard games that parents play," said one psychologist.

"If you study the bonding behaviors and attachment behaviors in the normal infant-mother development, you'll find that a lot of retarded kids lack the behavioral repertoire to assist in the bonding.

"So parents have to be aware that it is not their fault; that from birth, there's going to be a difficulty in bonding, and they have to be given some assistance to bond. Then they have to know that there's also going to be problems in separation and individuation.

"Professionals also need to know this. Often, you'll hear professionals saying that a parent is overprotecting their child, when in reality the parent is not overprotecting at all; the parent is responding to the child in terms of the child's emotional age rather than in terms of their chronological age, and the professionals often think the parents should be responding to their child in terms of their chronological age. The parents may know more about what their child needs than the professional, although there will always be some parents who go to extremes by overprotecting the child. We have to be careful of that.

"But we have to balance our view by considering those parents who are really responding to the child's emotional level rather than their chronological age. We need to help them with bonding. We need to let the parents know that the child is going to take longer to separate and individuate, and he's going to have more problems. The retarded child with motor problems can't crawl away from his mother and then crawl back quickly enough. He may crawl away; but when he gets too far from his mother, he'll become anxious because he can't crawl back fast enough, whereas the normal two-year-old comes and goes, comes and goes.

84 | A GUIDE TO MENTAL RETARDATION

"That's what the infant-stimulation programs should help parents with. I think they're fine with all the rehabilitation, physical therapies, and the language and speech development. The weak point of many early intervention programs is helping the parent and child in the emotional aspects of their relationship."

Finding the strength to cope involved finding strength not only within each parent but also within the family and family structure. Researchers have found that much of the previous literature on families overlooks the evidence that many families *do* cope with having a son or daughter with mental retardation (Summers, Behr, and Turnbull 1989).

All parents and all families have strengths to draw on in times of crisis and stress. The particular strengths will vary from parent to parent and family to family. Some families will be comforted and strengthened by their religious or ethical beliefs. Others will draw on support from each other and from extended family members. Still others will rely on friends, neighbors, or the support provided by parent support and advocacy. Some parents will benefit from professional counseling and support.

Families find many different ways to work together effectively. Some find it helpful to become involved in an early intervention program and various support groups. Other parents find that actually teaching their child some basic skills is a good way to feel some control over their situation.

The home teaching approach may be even more appropriate in situations where parents do not have access to an early intervention program, or the existing programs do not meet the needs of the family or of the child. Home teaching is not for everyone, but it is not necessarily complicated or time-consuming. There are a number of excellent books which clearly explain the teaching techniques, and are designed for use by parents and other family members (see, for example, Baker and Brightman 1989).

Perhaps the most important part of finding strength in the family is taking time to *look* for the strength in each parent and in the whole family. At a time of crisis and disruption, the temptation is to focus completely on problems and difficulties. It can take real effort and a lot of support to identify the coping resources in the family.

One parent gives the following words of wisdom: "I received two cards that were particularly meaningful to me. One was from close friends of ours who basically said: 'We have no idea what it is like. We just want you to know that we will be nearby and will try to learn with you.' That meant a lot to me, because no one knows what this is going to mean. You don't have any sense about what is going to happen. You have no sense that love will conquer all, that you'll be able to care for this child. That is not a feeling that I had. I did need reassurance, and I was reassured by someone saying, 'Hey, we'll see what happens.'

"The other things that was meaningful to me was something my aunt wrote in a letter. She said: 'As you grow older, you find that the line of certainty is very thin.' To me, this seemed real. The notion that 'youth, good intentions, sincerity, and kindness conquers all' may have truth, but it doesn't mean that you are going to be kept from tragedy and pain that will change your life forever.

"That seemed like what my feeling was: that this is going to change who we are. We are changed, and we will always be different. That seemed honest and forthright, like saying, 'God, no one ever said that I was never going to be healthy.'

"As each day goes by, you find a way to deal with it. The truth is that time does often let mending and healing happen. It was hard to feel that back then, but after a while I could sense that my hurt had changed.

"I also got a lot of strength from my wife who seems better to able to endure in many ways. So when I say how I am doing, it is a reflection of how we, as a couple, are coping, even if we don't know what we are going to do."

It is also easy to forget that a child with mental retardation makes a positive contribution to his or her family. According to another parent: "For most of the families I know, it's not a big deal that they have a child that is mentally retarded. They include their child in all their family activities.

"Most of us have found strength in having a child with mental retardation — there's no question about that. You find yourself more accepting of everyone; more accepting of all people with differences. I've heard parents say sincerely that it is the best thing that has ever happened to them."

When Mike talks about his child, he radiates the love he and his wife have for their son: "Steven is really a nice person. Very early on, there was a part of him that revealed to us this nice kid.

86 | A GUIDE TO MENTAL RETARDATION

He was a nice baby, and in many ways he made us feel that we had someone to take care of who was interesting. This helped us to be patient about who he was becoming."

Ann and Rud Turnbull are parents of a son with mental retardation and list the following positive family contributions that a child with mental retardation can make to the family: "Being a source of joy; providing a means of learning life's lessons; giving and receiving love; supplying a sense of blessing or fulfillment; contributing a source of pride; and strengthening a family" (1990, 115).

While many different people may offer their support and words of comfort, there are times when sincere efforts actually provide little nourishment for the emotional needs of the family. Mike explains: "I did not feel any sense of hope when people told me that I had been chosen; that I was to be a parent of a high-need child.

"Some people's religious tradition maintains that God doles out only what we are able to deal with. That is not my religious framework at all. I don't feel we were chosen by any God to do this. I think it was something that happened, and if God had his or her way, he would have chosen our child *not* to be retarded.

"At this point, I think I needed someone to say something wise, something that didn't imply that I was the savior for this child. I didn't want to be the savior. I wanted to care for my son in fun ways, sensible ways, and in terrible ways when I'm not doing well.

"There are things that happen in the course of the day that make me sad. I wish everyday that my son weren't retarded. I would like to know him without his having Down syndrome. I would like him to have experiences without his being retarded. As far as I can tell, I will always feel this way."

The emphasis on family coping and family strength is not meant to imply that families do not need the help and support of professionals and outside agencies. Rather, this emphasis on coping assumes that efforts to help and support the family will probably be more successful if these efforts are based on family strength and coping.

In the coping process it is important to keep in perspective the needs of the child with mental retardation, as well as the needs of all family members. While caring for a child with mental retardation will probably take considerable time and effort from all the family members, there has to be some consideration for the needs of all. Husbands and wives need time for each other, other children need the attention of parents, and family members will have other responsibilities in the extended family, the community, and employment that have nothing to do with mental retardation.

The most important task here is to strike a balance which recognizes the needs of each family member, but striking a balance does not mean that each family member gets *equal* time. It is important to be sure that the needs of one family member do not dominate the family energies to the exclusion of the needs of the others.

In order to keep this delicate balance, parents may need to prioritize and schedule their time. Needs and issues may need to be prioritized so they don't become so overwhelming and consuming. If needs and issues are not addressed, they will probably re-emerge and require attention, usually at the most inconvenient time.

Keeping a perspective includes keeping a sense of humor. The families that cope best have a good sense of humor and know that sometimes in life the only thing you can do is back off from a situation or problem and laugh about it.

The families most successful at coping find a way to work together so that, at one time or another, all the members of the family have their needs met. How this is accomplished varies greatly from family to family. Some families succeed by drawing on their own resources. Others draw on members of the extended family, friends, neighbors, and relatives. Still other family members make use of the support provided by professionals and agencies. Most families seem to find it beneficial to draw from many different sources in order to meet different needs.

The most important part of working together is for each family member to feel that he or she is important to the family, and that no family member is so totally involved in caring for the child with mental retardation that others are excluded, or that no one is so detached from the situation that he or she feels no responsibility to the family. How all this is worked out will vary from family to family, and even within families, from time to time, and situation to situation. Sometimes the family coping system will be

88 | A GUIDE TO MENTAL RETARDATION

freshly challenged by a crisis; but with appropriate support from inside and/or outside of the family, the family members are usually able to start working together again. There is no one best way to cope with or care for a young child with a handicapping condition, but most families, in spite of many problems and struggles, manage to provide a loving home.

3

School and the Child with Mental Retardation

"What goes on in a self-contained classroom?"

Legislation

In 1975, the United States Congress passed P.L. 94–142, **The Education for All Handicapped Children Act**, affecting the education of every child with mental retardation in the United States. The intent of P.L. 94–142 is to provide the funds for a free, appropriate education to every child with mental retardation or other handicapping condition. The goal of the law is to prepare students with handicaps to live as independently as possible as adults.

Perhaps one of the most radical assumptions behind P.L. 94–142 is that all children, no matter how severe their disabilities, could benefit from an appropriate education. Another assumption is that most students with mental retardation and other handicaps can be educated in their local community schools with nonhandicapped children.

Based on previous federal legislation, this was clearly the first law to spell out the rights of students with mental retardation to participate fully in the public education system in the United States.

90 | A GUIDE TO MENTAL RETARDATION

Requirements of P.L. 94–142

P.L. 94–142 is a complex legislation in which Congress clearly defines how a student with mental retardation should be educated. Some of the major provisions of this law include:

(a) The right to a free, appropriate education at public expense for all students, no matter how severe their handicap;

(b) A complete evaluation of the specific needs of each student, and the development of an educational program to address those specific needs. This educational program must be documented for each student in an Individualized Education Program (IEP);

(c) The IEP will be revised and evaluated at least annually, and it will include measurable goals and objectives to evaluate student progress;

(d) If a student in need of special education requires certain related services (that is, transportation, physical or occupational therapy, speech and language therapy, specialized equipment, counseling and social work) in order to meet educational goals, these services must be provided at no expense to the student or to his or her parents;

(e) The student in need of special education will be educated in the Least Restrictive Environment (LRE) which permits that student to attain his or her educational goals. For most students with mental retardation, the LRE will be the special education program in the local public school.

P.L. 94–142 does *not* mandate that all students in special education be educated along with nonhandicapped students of the same age. Rather, the legislation requires that the particular student's unique educational needs be taken into account when designating the LRE.

(f) P.L. 94–142 clearly defines the rights of the parents of a student in special education or being assessed for special education. These include the right of the parents to be informed and to participate in the design of their child's IEP, the right to confidentiality of information regarding their child, and a process for the appeal of educational decisions that parents feel are not in their child's best interest.

(g) The student's IEP will be developed by an interdisciplinary team consisting of special education teachers, representatives of the school administration, parents, and other professionals (for example, physical therapists, speech and language therapists).

Other Legislation: P.L. 101–476

The rights of students with mental retardation to an appropriate education at public expense were reconfirmed when the Individuals with Disabilities Education Act (P.L. 101–476) was signed into law in 1990. This act confirmed the requirements of P.L. 94–142, and expanded the requirements in some areas. The new legislation provides funding for additional services, equipment, and training in the area of assistive technology or equipment which enables a student to function more independently.

It should be noted that this part of the legislation only refers to equipment and technology to help a student attain a goal on his or her IEP; it does not provide for the purchase of equipment which is not related to an educational goal. Secondly, if a school district purchases equipment for a student, that equipment usually remains the property of the district after the student has achieved his or her educational goal, or after the student is no longer covered by the special education law — usually age twenty-one or twenty-two — or if the student leaves the district.

Another important provision of P.L. 101–476 is the emphasis on transition services. These services are used to help a student move from one educational setting to another, or from school to the adult world. The new legislation requires that the IEP of all students have a transition plan for services by the age of sixteen, at the latest. These transition plans are usually designed to help a student develop employment skills and the ability to live as independently as possible as an adult.

There are a number of other important provisions of P.L. 101–476 which may affect some students with mental retardation. The new legislation adds funding for services directed toward infants and toddlers with multiple handicaps, and increases funding for some programs for students who are deaf and blind. Some students with mental retardation will be in this category.

P.L. 101–476 specifically includes autism as a handicapping condition for the first time under federal law, although autism had already been included in a number of previous state laws. There is considerable overlap between autism and mental retardation (see Gerdtz and Bregman 1990).

The Rights of Parents: P.L. 99–372

Another important federal law for parents of students in special education is the Handicapped Children's Protection Act of 1986 (P.L. 99–372). This law allows parents and guardians to recover attorney's fees from court actions and administrative hearings, under certain conditions.

First, the parents or guardians must prevail (or "win") in the court action or administrative hearing. Second, the legal fees must be reasonable. Third, the parents must have acted in good faith. Accordingly, parents who reject a compromise offered by the school system which the court feels was a reasonable offer will not receive attorney's fees.

There are also provisions in the law to reduce the amount of attorney's fees to be recovered in certain circumstances (Florian and West 1989). This law is intended to give parents the ability to challenge inappropriate decisions in the special education system, while at the same time encouraging reasonable compromise between parents and school districts, as well as discouraging unnecessary litigation.

While parents have an extensive appeals process available to them, less than 1% of the parents involved in special education have used the appeals process (Florian and West 1989, 7). This may mean that the vast majority of parents are satisfied with the services their child receives through the special education system, or that many parents are not aware of their rights. Other parents may be intimidated by the complexity of the appeals process.

Studies of administrative fair hearings in special education found that in order to prevail in most of these hearings parents or their attorneys must be able to present considerable evidence, produce witnesses, and cross-examine the witnesses of the school district (Goldberg and Kuriloff 1991).

Surveys of both parents and school district officials indicate that even families who win court cases and administrative hearings in special education find the process exhausting and disheartening (Goldberg and Kuriloff 1991). Still those with the most negative experiences in the appeals system seem to feel that the system was necessary to protect students in special education.

Parents and special education professionals need to be reasonable and open to appropriate compromises when disputes arise around a student's IEP. At the same time, parents need to be aware of their rights in the appeals process, and be ready to use the process if necessary, in order to obtain the best possible education for their son or daughter with mental retardation.

Legislation has made it possible for a large number of children with mental retardation to receive a good education in their local schools. However, a number of problems result from misunderstanding the legislation. For example, some parents and advocates have difficulty understanding that the legislation guarantees an appropriate education to a student with a handicap, but this does not mean that the student is entitled at public expense to the best possible education. Generally, the courts have agreed that the education provided must address the goals of the student's IEP, but the education does not have to be the best that money can buy, or the type of education that experts would design for children with mental retardation.

Professionals, too, have their misunderstandings. In spite of the very small number of actual court cases and administrative hearings actually brought by parents, there is a perception among some professionals that "parents have all the rights" under the legislation.

The legislation makes a strong statement about the rights of parents, but at the same time it attempts to encourage compromise between parents and professionals, and discourage unnecessary litigation. Much of this same legislation also provides funds for the training of professionals in special education and related disciplines.

Another problem area for special education legislation and funding is in the perception of parents of nonhandicapped children, and of teachers and administrators in the regular education system. For example, with recent severe budget cuts in many school districts, a number of parents and school district administrators have complained about the high cost of special education, and the level of services provided to students in special education.

94 | A GUIDE TO MENTAL RETARDATION

It is true that special education is expensive, and the average student in special education generally will have more funds spent on his or her education than a nonhandicapped peer.

A nationwide study of the costs of special education (Kakalik, Furry, Thomas, and Carney 1981) found that special education costs more than twice as much per pupil than regular education. It is also true that special education programs, in general, have not had the severe budget cuts many regular education programs have had.

Parents and professionals in special education face the on-going challenge of making the general community aware of the need for special education and the benefits that special education provides to the community at large.

Those of us involved in special education should also be supportive of regular education, and the need for a good educational system for all the children in a community. We need to make the best use of the funds and resources we have, and to develop effective educational programs. Good special education does not have to be expensive. Research has shown that many of the most effective techniques in special education could be introduced at relatively low cost.

Another misunderstanding in special education is due to a false assumption made by many parents and professionals in the field that adults with mental retardation and other handicapping conditions are guaranteed programs similar to those they received as school-age children.

The truth is that special education legislation covers toddlers, preschoolers, and school-age children, but does not apply to those over the age of twenty-one or twenty-two. Parents are often surprised and angered to discover that their son or daughter, now an adult, is not entitled to any specific service. And while most communities have programs for adults with mental retardation, these programs are often full and have waiting lists.

It is extremely important for parents and professionals to plan ahead — at least five or six years — to help a student with mental retardation make a successful transition to adult programs. Parents should make themselves familiar with the adult programs in their community while their son or daughter is still in school, and determine which programs and services may or may not be available.

It may also be necessary to form alliances with other parents, develop relationships with adult service programs, and lobby politicians and others for services which may not currently be available. It may take years to develop programs even after funding has been approved, so it is important to lay the groundwork for these programs before a child finishes school and is no longer eligible for services through the school system.

What Is Good Special Education?

The following characteristics of a good education for students with mental retardation have been adapted from the best practice guidelines developed by the Center for Development Disabilities at the University of Vermont (1987).

The major characteristics of a good special education include: (1) partnership with parents; (2) opportunity for the student to interact with nonhandicapped students; (3) opportunity for the student to participate in community settings; (4) curriculum; (5) systematic instruction; (6) transition planning; (7) regular evaluation of services; and (8) individualized student assessment and educational techniques.

Partnership with Parents

Good special education is carried out in partnership with parents. Legislation requires programs to keep parents informed through the Individualized Education Plan (IEP) process, but effective programs offer parents more opportunity to be involved — with suggestions for carrying out educational goals and objectives at home, communication through a daily or weekly log book, parent meetings or newsletters, and other practices.

Parents can reinforce the special education program by continuing some parts of the program at home whenever possible. Another role parents can play in the partnership, and one that should never be underestimated, is to show support and appreciation to teachers and other staff.

Opportunity to Interact with Nonhandicapped Students

The opportunity for students with mental retardation to have regular contact and interaction with other students of the same age range is an important part of the educational process. This is best

96 | A GUIDE TO MENTAL RETARDATION

achieved if the special education program is located in a local public school.

Even if the special education program is located in a setting away from the public school, the teacher and other staff should be encouraged to find opportunities for students with mental retardation to work together with nonhandicapped students. This might be achieved by developing a program where nonhandicapped students act as peer tutors for the students in special education, or programs in which students in special education and nonhandicapped students work together on some common project to benefit the community.

One parent agrees: "The ideal situation, from my viewpoint, is for a handicapped child to participate in a class with nonhandicapped children of the same age.

"Of course there's no way I would expect the handicapped child to do the same work as twenty-seven nonhandicapped kids the same age. Let's say we're in fourth grade: those twenty-seven nonhandicapped kids will be doing the regular fourth-grade curriculum, as they should. Now you have a child with mental retardation who is nine years old, like the other kids, but who obviously won't be able to do the fourth-grade work. But that child has an IEP — an Individualized Education Plan; he should be working toward the goals on his IEP, while the other kids are working toward the regular, fourth-grade curriculum goals.

"There may be a few places where they can overlap — like in music, art, or gym. But I wouldn't expect the nine-year-old with mental retardation to be doing long multiplication like the other fourth graders. But while they're doing multiplication during arithmetic, maybe the kid with mental retardation is doing subtraction or addition. He'd be doing math at the same time they're doing math, but not the same work.

"You also would develop a lot of peer tutoring to help out. In the meantime, those twenty-seven kids realize that, 'Hey, here's a handicapped child the same age as us. He's not capable of doing the same work as us, but that's okay. He has limitations — fine. He is still our friend. He is still our buddy. We're going to help him. We're going to play with him. We're going to be his friends.'

"So now the self-esteem of that handicapped child rises. Not only that, the self-esteem of some of the twenty-seven other kids will also go up. But out of those twenty-seven kids, there's probably five or six who, themselves, are having difficulty with their academic work for one reason or another. If they are able to peer tutor a kid who is mentally retarded, their own self-esteem will go up. And you learn something better when you teach it to someone else.

"The ideal situation is to have handicapped kids mingle with regular kids in a natural proportion, which would be about 10:1. (Ten to twelve percent of the population in the United States. is handicapped.) So you figure if you have thirty kids in a classroom, maybe three of them are going to be kids with a handicap — learning disability or whatever. This is ideal."

Opportunity to Participate in Community Settings

If students with mental retardation are to learn to be as independent and self-sufficient as possible when they are adults, they must have the opportunity to develop and practice these skills in a number of different community settings. The community settings will range from stores and restaurants to part-time job sites and local recreational facilities.

Interacting with nonhandicapped students and participating in community settings help the individual develop social skills which are the essential foundation for successful and independent life in the community for adults with mental retardation, and are especially important in maintaining employment (McLoughlin, Garner, and Callahan 1987).

The importance of integrating handicapped children into the mainstream is clear. One parent expressed his concern over his son's opportunity to make friends with the neighborhood kids, and his feeling that segregating mentally retarded children only disrupts this possibility: "While parents are concerned about their child receiving the best education appropriate for their child's needs, a greater concern is for their child to interact with his or her peers. Schools are a place where kids learn socialization skills.

"We want our kids to develop friendships and become part of society. But first, they need to become part of the school community. What they learn academically is only a part of their education and not necessarily the most important part.

"This is why it is so important to us that our kids go to school with their siblings and the kids from their neighborhood. When

98 | A GUIDE TO MENTAL RETARDATION

the child goes to another school on the other side of the county or town, it is very hard for that child to develop friendships in the neighborhood.

"To make matters worse, the children in a class that comes from all parts of the county can't develop friendships with classmates because they don't live near them. And when they come home on the school bus, they try to play with the neighborhood kids, but they don't know them because they didn't see each other in school all day. It becomes very hard to establish friendships.

"When a kid is six years old that may not be a big problem; [kids that age] spend a lot of time in their house anyway. But when a child is thirteen, and comes home from school and doesn't have any friends to play with — now, that's a problem.

"Just because a kid is retarded doesn't mean he's not lonely. These kids are smart enough to know when they don't have any friends. Their self-esteem goes down, and it's just going to make matters worse.

"This is why we say a separate education system is not an equal education system. To sum it up, I feel that the educational needs of any special child can, and should be, met in his or her home school with as much interaction with nonhandicapped peers as possible — or as appropriate, or a combination of the two. There is no reason why you can't meet special educational needs in that home school."

If the child with mental retardation is not allowed to interact with his or her nonhandicapped peers, some believe these individuals will not be able to develop the social skills necessary to live a successful and independent life in the community as adults.

One parent talks about his position on inclusion: "The dream I have for my son when he turns twenty-two is not that he's going to live in a group home — although I have nothing against group homes, they're a hundred times better than institutions — but I see group homes as a temporary thing; I hope twenty years from now there aren't any group homes.

"I have this dream that a couple of young men come up to me and say, 'We want your son to live with us; not because we're being paid to do it, but because your son is our friend and we know he needs a place to live.' But those two young men will never exist unless they've gone through school with kids like my son.

"If we don't get things changed around in the schools, every-thing else will go down the tubes. Kids who are retarded are going to grow up and face the same problems retarded people do today. Some of them are going to be lucky enough to get jobs in real places with job coaches. But a lot of them won't; they're going to wind up working in workshops.

"For a lot of retarded adults today, their life *is* the workshop. Then they go home to the group home. Their social life involves other retarded people — they go bowling, they go to dances, all with their little group of retarded people. But they don't have friends who aren't handicapped. To me, that's the worse thing. What kind of life is that?"

Curriculum

In good special education, the curriculum guides staff and parents as to what skills and tasks are important, how to assess a student, how to evaluate student progress, and where to go next after a student has mastered a task. Some teachers and programs are effective at developing their own curriculum, while others find it helpful to make use of a curriculum developed for another program, or one available commercially.

A further advantage of a good comprehensive curriculum is that by using the curriculum the teacher will address many of the characteristics of effective educational programs in the areas of assessment, data collection, systematic evaluation of student progress, and so on.

Systematic Instruction

Good special education requires the use of a variety of teaching techniques. The interested reader should consult articles reviewing these techniques (for example, Ault, Wolery, Doyle, and Gast 1989).

Most parents will not be familiar with teaching procedures, but all effective procedures require some form of regular data collec-tion. It seems that, to be effective, data collection should be done daily or weekly, and certainly no less frequently than every month. Unfortunately, research on special education classrooms indicates that data collection is often no more frequent than once a

100 | A GUIDE TO MENTAL RETARDATION

year, which is virtually useless in monitoring student progress (Zigmond and Miller 1986).

The most effective type of data collection involves daily measurement of student progress on important goals and objectives; graphing data helps teachers make more accurate predictions of student progress (Marston 1988, 38–39). Naturally, it is no use collecting data if the information is not used to assess student progress and to make changes in educational and training programs as needed.

Ironically, research indicates that special education teachers who do not make use of frequent data collection and evaluation are more optimistic about student goal attainment than teachers who keep and use systematic data-collection procedures (Fuchs, Fuchs, and Stecker 1989). Of course, the optimism of those who may not know what they are talking about will be of cold comfort to most parents.

Being a good special education teacher is both an art and a science. The science part involves systematic teaching techniques, data collection, and evaluation and is very important. Equally important is the art of teaching. In addition, good teachers manage to show parents, students, and other staff that they care about their students and expect the students to learn.

Transition Planning

Good special education includes preparing a student for adulthood. It is crucial that this planning start early enough for the student to develop social and other skills necessary to function as independently as possible in the community. This may result in the student's being involved in a work-study program in the last few years of high school in order to develop and sharpen employment skills. Frequent exposure to community settings such as stores, restaurants, and recreation programs, along with systematic instruction in appropriate behavior in these settings, will help a student cultivate skills and abilities needed to function as independently as possible as an adult.

The transition planning process should begin no later than age sixteen, and earlier if possible. Parents and current special education staff should meet, with a representative of the adult service system if possible. The transition plan should be specific and focused on those skills and needs (for example, employment, independent living) which would help this particular individual live as independently as possible in the community.

Regular Evaluation of Services

Just as the progress of students in special education should be monitored on a regular basis in order to assess student progress, the staff of the special education program should evaluate the program to determine if the program is performing as effectively and efficiently as possible.

Part of this regular program assessment should be an evaluation of the satisfaction of parents with the program, the morale of the special education staff, the program's compliance with regulations and best practices in the field of special education, monitoring of gains in student progress, and the success of individuals who have completed the program.

The goal of this type of program evaluation is not simply to indicate potential problems, although this should be an important part of the process. The evaluation should be structured to indicate successes as well, and should be part of an ongoing system of program evaluation and change. Parents should also try to use a program evaluation not only as a time to highlight problems, but also to indicate areas in which the program has been successful for their son or daughter.

Individualized Assessment and Teaching

In many ways, this is the core of effective special education, and is clearly mandated by federal and state regulations. There is generally confusion as to the role of individualization with all the previous discussion of structured teaching techniques, curricula, and data collection. In fact, there need be no conflict at all among these characteristics. While where is a core of effective teaching techniques and procedures for students with mental retardation, these techniques are most effective when used in accordance with a particular student's needs and strengths.

This is why regular assessment of students and student progress is so important. Some students will respond to one teaching technique; other students will respond more effectively to other techniques. A good assessment will make clear a student's

102 | A GUIDE TO MENTAL RETARDATION

correct strengths and needs, and will indicate priorities for instruction and training.

This is not to imply that classroom instruction can, or should, be totally individual. Students with mental retardation will need to be able to learn in groups, and be able to contribute to the completion of group projects. Most of the effective teaching techniques will be effective with only a number of students. But it is essential that the special education staff have a good understanding of the individual needs of each student. If parents find that all students in a classroom have exactly the same goals and objectives, it is likely that assessment and instruction is appropriately individualized.

If a parent has an understanding of special education legislation, as well as the general principles of good teaching in special education, that parent will be able to judge, to some extent, whether his or her child is receiving a good special education.

Children with mental retardation who are of school age have, by virtue of federal and state legislation, the opportunity to receive intensive educational services at public expense. As noted above, adults with mental retardation are not entitled to the same level of services. So it is essential that parents, special education teachers and staff, and students with mental retardation make the best use of educational opportunities available during the school years.

More on Inclusion — Different Views

One professional expressed his concerns: "The bigger issue is: Will kids be mainstreamed? Or will they always have to be in a special class somewhere in the wing of their building? The answer is — Yes: there will always be some kids who will have to be in a special class, isolated somewhere in their building. Those kids — when talking about the developmentally disabled — will probably be the more aggressive.

"The real conflict is going to come with this *inclusion* notion — assuming that you can take a nonaggressive, ten-year-old retarded child with a mental age of five and put him in a class with normal ten-year-olds at the fifth-grade level, and assume that he's going to learn something under these conditions. I don't think this is going to work.

School and the Child with Mental Retardation | 103

"This has actually started now. There are some retarded kids being mainstreamed — it's called *inclusion* rather than mainstreamed — and they are actually sitting in a fifth-grade class, being exposed to fifth-grade materials. There's one retarded child I know in a fifth-grade class who can't even read.

"Personally, I don't understand how they're going to learn anything under those conditions. Maybe I'm old-fashioned. Maybe they will find a way where they'll be able to something. But I don't know if that is truly inclusion just to sit there.

"I think it's a denial that the handicapped are different. Do you think that the ten-year-old children are going to play with this ten-year-old retarded child after school? Of course not!

"So parents are going to be left with trying to find peers for their ten-year-old child with a mental age of five; the kids in his class aren't going to play with him. It's not true that a normal ten-year-old is going to play with a same-aged child with a mental age of five.

"I think the concept of inclusion and mainstreaming will have the adverse effect of isolating the handicapped child from the friendships he could potentially have with youngsters of the same mental age.

"Now if someone said to put this child in with five-year-olds — children of the same mental age — I would probably buy that first; I'm not sure how it would work out, but I would accept that model before I would accept the concept of inclusion. I've seen five-year-olds play with adults having a mental age of five; the adult gets down on the floor and plays with them just like a five-year-old. I think there's a greater potential for this to happen.

"Nothing — not even the concept of inclusion — is recent. We keep reinventing the wheel. Years ago, in the one-room schoolhouses, the 'retarded' children were educated in the mainstream; and the reason they were removed from that mainstream was that they weren't learning.

"Now we're saying the reason they were removed from the mainstream was society's prejudice; society didn't accept the handicapped. It's actually not true, if you really know the history of this field. The original founders of the institutions for the mentally retarded really felt they could make a major impact on by grouping them together. They found, however, that they couldn't make the impact they wanted to make.

104 | A GUIDE TO MENTAL RETARDATION

"There was this hope that society could make the individual with mental retardation 'normal' by creating the right environment, the right instruction. They certainly did have some impact — they educated individuals to their potential. The key is that we educated individuals to their potential, but we weren't satisfied with that. We wanted to educate them to some mythical potential that they could never reach."

A school psychologist talks about what individuals with mental retardation feel about mainstreaming: "We know from formal academic research that the individual can get depressed, that he or she is aware that he or she is different.

"But I don't think we've done enough work. In the first place, it's hard to do work like this. For example, if you take the I.Q. range of 55 to 89, and these people disappear into the community and they're never again labeled 'mentally retarded' — they're only labeled when they are in the schools — it's very hard to follow them, to find out how they feel looking back on their childhood.

"What we generally find, asking these people if they liked being in special classes, is that they say, 'Of course not. I hated being in the special class. I wanted to be in the mainstream.' But if you asked those who had been in the mainstream before we had special classes, they will tell you that their lives were miserable, that they were subjected to teasing; they were far behind in class, they didn't know who to play with — the kids wouldn't play with them after school, they ignored them in class.

"So often the child didn't have a choice. A bunch of them grew up being in the mainstream before we had special classes and they felt miserable about being different. Then a bunch of them, when we put them into special classes, felt miserable about being different. But at least they had some peers that were there so that they could form some friendships and that parents could arrange for activities after school.

"In general, follow-up of those clients with I.Q.s above 55 who are out in the work force hasn't told us what is the best kind of approach for them. I don't think we've asked clients with I.Q.s below 55 these questions either; they have a hard time expressing themselves.

"They have asked a few clients from a developmental center how they like being in the group home, and the responses were mixed: Some liked it better in the institution, and some like it better in the group homes. It could depend upon a lot of things including previous programs they attended, or friendships that may have been broken up — it's very hard for the individual with mental retardation to make friends."

Parents and Their Prejudices

An administrator talks about her dealings with families: "It's tough for us — and for me, speaking personally — to really see where this issue is going to go. We've had some interesting conversations here about the prejudices of some parents with children with handicapping conditions toward other children with handicapping conditions.

"These families who are so intent on having their child involved in services offering an inclusionary setting are very nearly discriminating against other handicapped kids. They are saying things like, 'I don't want my child with those handicapped kids,' or with children who have a particular type of handicapping condition. It's like saying, 'I want my child with speech- and language-delayed children, but not with an autistic child who may be flapping his arms for self-stimulation.' Or they may say, 'Don't put my Down syndrome child with an autistic child.' "

The Media and the Public Image of Mental Retardation

"I recall watching an episode from a television series the other night," recalls a program director. "In it was one of the more well-known Down syndrome children, Jason Kingsley — whose mother, Emily Kingsley, is a writer for Sesame Street. (Jason has been in movies, and has been on Sesame Street himself as a young child.) Along with Jason on the show was his friend, another person with Down syndrome. After watching this show, I wondered if parents of children with Down syndrome saw this show differently from how I did.

"One image presented was that Jason's best friends are other people with developmental disabilities, which is a very accurate image of the way things are today. Sure, he went to school with normal kids, and he was in regular education classes with normal kids; but when it came down to who he socialized with outside of school, it was other people with disabilities. The main character even went to the prom with another girl with Down syndrome. In

106 | A GUIDE TO MENTAL RETARDATION

general, I feel that this is okay; it is all right to try and accept the situation as it is.

"I'm afraid that parents of children with disabilities don't think this is good enough. I think the parents, instead, should be thrilled and excited that their child went to a prom! Does it matter who they went with?"

A special education teacher talks about some of the pressure parents feel: "I have had a relatively new parent of a child with Down syndrome — maybe a two-year-old child — pull me aside and ask, 'If he's not walking now, does that mean he will be one of those *lower functioning* Down syndrome children when he's older?' Again, that's when we start talking about *now*. It's upsetting to see them comparing. A lot of times they do bring up these skewed images from television and the media. It is a pressure. It really feels, in some ways, a pressure that they need to have the *perfect* handicapped child.

"I had a conversation last night with a special education teacher who has a class of children with learning disabilities, and next year she's moving her kids into a fourth-grade *team-teaching* situation.

"I was relieved to hear that a district was responding at that level. It seemed to me that that should have taken place way before some of these other steps. If you're going to try to acclimate regular education staff to dealing with kids with disabilities in their classroom, let's start with more mildly impaired kids and work them in before we throw in a more severely impaired kid."

* * *

The remainder of this chapter is an article written by Michaela D'Aquanni, a special education teacher at LaGrange Elementary School in LaGrange, New York. Ms. D'Aquanni wrote this article for the 1990 edition of *Perceptions,* the newsletter of the New York State Association of Special Educators. The article is reprinted here with permission.

School and the Child with Mental Retardation | 107

It's Time To Mix, Not Match

After reviewing the history of the development, education, and acceptance of people with special needs in our society, we need to hope that the future will speak better of us. Until recently, parents who gave birth to a child with a handicapping condition were painted a bleak picture of hopelessness and given a list of institutions in which to place their child. "Tell the relatives the baby is dead" — out of sight, out of mind. This was an expected route, as if removing people with handicapping conditions from society would remove the handicap. Today, if you seek out trained and knowledgeable professionals, you may instead be given hope and a smile, lists of early intervention programs, and leave feeling that your child's life has value and will be as productive as anyone else's.

Because education and knowledge can help, we need to focus on the education of the general population as well as the education of people with special needs. Since the passage of the Education for All Handicapped Children Act (P.L. 94–142) in 1975, many changes have occurred. The law states that

> To the maximum extent appropriate, handicapped children [are to be] educated with children who are not handicapped. Special classes, separate schooling, or other removal from the regular education environment occurs only when the nature of the severity of the handicap is such that education in regular classes with use of supplementary aids and services cannot be achieved satisfactorily.

As clear as this may seem, the interpretation of the law has led to many different outcomes. Although prepared definitions have been forwarded to all schools to use for identifying children with special needs, a child labeled in one school may be completely overlooked in another. In one situation, you may have severely handicapped students working side-by-side with their nonhandicapped peers, while in the next district, handicapped students are housed in self-contained classes or even [in a] self-contained school.

108 | A GUIDE TO MENTAL RETARDATION

Children who look or act the same do not necessarily have the same abilities. Children who achieve at the same levels or score the same on achievement tests do not necessarily have the same abilities either. So why then do we continue to match students according to their predetermined abilities instead of mixing them and allowing them to learn from each other's abilities: Is it possible that we judge people more by what they cannot do than by what they can do? Maybe it is time we started looking for the solution instead of always looking for the problem.

Recent research has shown that Down syndrome children are not all alike . . . that most are only mildly retarded and a few can even reach normal levels of intelligence. . . . In many instances their retardation is as much the product of low expectations, understimulation, and lack of education as it is a product of a genetic defect (Turkington 1987, 42, 44). . . . Many early childhood books tell us that children learn best through imitation, modeling, and peer influence. So why then do we continue to put all the language-delayed children in one room, all the [children with] behavior problems . . . in another, all the "different learners" in another room, etc.? We need to remember basic theories of early childhood education when we place children in least restrictive and appropriate educational environments.

I think it would be valuable for us to start removing obstacles that separate students with special needs from their peers as well as special education teachers from their colleagues. A current philosophy fostered by P.L. 94–142 is that of integration. As educators we can no longer focus on educating persons, no matter what their ability, with two schools of education: regular and special. Special education is supposed to support regular education, not be a separate entity. Although thought of as a magic place where children go to get "fixed," special education uses no special methods or materials. The needs of special education teachers are the same as regular education teachers: to use appropriate and effective teaching models for all students and to be caring and loving. Rather than researching where it all went wrong, we need to focus on how to bring things back — not to where they once were, but to a more congenial, inclusive, and honorable way of teaching.

Integration, as I define it, is a process in which each child goes to the home school and participates in a regular class with age-appropriate peers, so that children can grow to the best of their ability, but not necessarily to the same degree as their peers. It provides a supportive environment in which children with special needs can play and grow with, as well as learn from, other youngsters. This disqualifies the need for children . . . to be transported on long bus rides to special classes away from their home schools. It also removes the need for failure and retentions. The teacher is the key to promoting success and continuous progress.

Our purse strings would not be pulled so tight, as we would have one uniform means of education and not two. Staff energy would be focused more on instruction and less on referrals and classification. If a child is in need of support services, these services should be provided in the classroom to the maximum extent possible. Remember, special education is a service and not a place. Regular students with need for extra support or instruction can also benefit from the influx of services in the classroom. Mainstreaming should not only be used as an excuse to start placing children in regular classrooms — that is where they belong to begin with.

Whatever age children are, and no matter what special needs they have, they still have a very common need for friendship and acceptance. One important point we need to emphasize is that of socialization. Children can acquire social as well as academic skills in school, including proper behavior, social etiquette, friendship, and the ability to interact. Students who are labeled handicapped are more alike than different from their peers. All children have the same basic needs: "To belong, to be affirmed, to be successful, and to serve" (DiFrancesco 1989). If these basic needs are not fulfilled, then the ability to learn is greatly impaired. Children with disabilities have the right "to go to school with their nondisabled peers, and their teacher should have learned how to take care of their special needs and to include them in all school activities. They also have the right to have the opportunity for education and training that they need in order to prepare themselves to work and to live independently" (Helander 1984, 23). . . .

Research supports the rights and needs of people with special needs by showing clearly that "maladaptive behavior diminishes when handicapped children are integrated with nonhandicapped. [Individuals with mental retardation] imitate the good behavior of

110 | A GUIDE TO MENTAL RETARDATION

their nonhandicapped peers and become better accepted by them. They develop faster and achieve better results. Nonhandicapped children also gain from the increased contact and integration with handicapped children" (World Health 1984, 19). However, we must take into consideration that attitudes are formed early in life; therefore, the sooner people are introduced to the broad range of individual differences, the more likely they will be to develop mutual understanding, tolerance, and respect for each other.

The attitudes of students, parents, teachers, and administrators all play a large role in the integration of the handicapped into present-day regular education programs. Young children, who have not yet formed attitudes, can be influenced as long as integration starts during the early years; it then becomes a way of life and is not perceived as anything different. Older children, who have never had contact with disabled children, have a more difficult time with an integrated school program. How many of us tend to stare, feel uncomfortable, and wonder "why" when we see a person with a disability? The only way to overcome these feelings of fear and uneasiness is to learn more about "why" and what these people are all about. Integration allows this teaming process to occur through real-life experiences, the most effective teaching tools. As one special friend put it, "Once you've worked with handicapped students for a while, they get to be just like normal friends. They're just regular people" (Hanline 1984, 274).

Parents of children with handicapping conditions are also caught in a struggle between enrolling their child in self-contained programs where they are "protected" and "safe" as compared to integrated programs where they have proper models and peer interaction to teach them about real-life situations, both pleasant and unpleasant. It is necessary to look to the future. Which situation would motivate and qualify individuals to lead a more independent life as well as better equip them to deal with the different attitudes of society? Parents must be prepared to help children deal with their anxieties, build their self-esteem, and feel they do not have to constantly compare themselves with their peers. Even for people with disabilities, "it is not whether you win or lose but how you play the game."

How amenable administrators and teachers are to integrating handicapped youngsters depends on their receptivity to change, how they handle present conflicts and relationships, and yes, their attitudes toward people with disabilities. Like anything new and untried, integration can create anxiety for all involved. Regular teachers are justified in their fears, as working with children with handicapping conditions is an unknown to them; however, rather than being frightened and keeping their distance, they should open themselves up to the idea and make adjustments. They need to build their confidence in their ability to teach children with disabilities. Teachers and administrators need to remember that their attitude will set the tone for the entire class. Their actions should display the feeling that every student is special.

When the educational system has joined forces — when regular and special education staff have formed new partnerships — it will be time to prepare a plan for complete integration. One should keep in mind two ideas: it is not going to happen overnight, and we must deal with many attitudes, some that are just forming and some that have been around for a while. Integration is not simply placing a child in a classroom without help for the regular classroom teachers. In-service training is a "must" for all teachers to adequately prepare for their newly assigned roles. Teachers need to develop positive attitudes toward the integration of children with special needs and develop knowledge, skills, and competent instructional methods for educating all students together. . . .

Students also need to be made knowledgeable about handicapping conditions and be prepared to accept those with special needs before the students enter the program. Most of us have seen the teasing, avoidance, and ridicule brought on by ignorance when the special education class walks down the hall. Some materials to deal with integration would be books, movies, plays, puppets (namely "The Kids on the Block," a company located in Washington, D.C., or "New Friends," an outreach program in Chapel Hill, North Carolina). Puppets are generally nonthreatening and can help initiate discussions that will promote understanding of people with handicapping conditions. Guest speakers who can discuss their disabilities can break down the walls of ignorance. Some teaching methods that would help teachers in the classroom are cooperative learning, curriculum adaptations, team-teaching, teaching through all modalities, class-wide peer tutoring, and be-

112 | A GUIDE TO MENTAL RETARDATION

havior support plans. Teachers should encourage children to think of themselves as "members of a support team with just two guidelines: to be friendly and to be themselves" (*Instructor Staff* 1989, 62). A lesson all children need to learn is to be able to put themselves in another person's shoes.

The success of an integrated program depends on the readiness of peers, teachers, administrators, parents, and other support staff. If problems arise during the process, a plan for problem-solving needs to be put into action. Communication is a key ingredient. In preparing the groundwork for integration, we need to remember that integration is NOT:

> " — a dumping ground into regular classes
> — trading off quality for integration
> — cutting back on special services
> — ignoring each child's needs
> — all learning the same way at the same time
> — expecting regular education teachers to teach without needed support
> — sacrificing education of regular children."
>
> (Schaffner et al. 1988, 9)

As we continue along the lines of integrating all people into society, let us remember that "all human beings should be considered of inherently equal worth. We are all born each a unique individual; each developing along different lines; each has different abilities. These differences do not make us unequal in worth."

Michaela D'Aquanni

4

Transition into Adulthood

A Time of Change

For the individual with a handicap, the twenty-first year marks a significant transition. It is a time when he or she is faced with leaving the familiarity of childhood — the teachers and friends from public school or from a special education program — to begin the process of living and working as an adult to the best of his or her ability.

This transitional period, often referred to as a time of "aging-out," becomes a significant and often stressful time, not only for the person with the developmental disability, but for the people who are involved with him or her as well. Out of concern for their child's future, parents make plans for continued programming and often face many stressors in their search.

Even before this transitional period, the life of an individual with a developmental disability has contained many different periods of emotional turmoil. Workers in the field describe these periods of developmental crisis as centering around experiences of loss, anxiety over incomplete mastery, and the need to develop greater autonomy; but while these stressful periods or "psychosocial milestones" are in every way similar to those experienced by the nonretarded, "the impact of developmental delays makes their resolution especially difficult for the mentally retarded and their family" (Gilson and Levitas 1987).

114 | A GUIDE TO MENTAL RETARDATION

The disabled child is sensitive to the overprotection of his or her parents which, in turn, may have intensified the child's own ambivalence about his or her own developing autonomy. With the arrival of brothers or sisters, the child is sensitive to the loss of attention he or she needs, and as a result may regress in functioning and behavior.

Starting school is the child's first prolonged experience away from the protection of the family. It can be a time when friendships with other children may come to an end as his or her social skills fall behind those of his or her peers and his or her cognitive abilities reach a plateau. Further milestones include the onset of puberty and adolescence; the feelings of discouragement and sadness when exposed to the issue of sex and dating; facing one's own limitations as younger siblings surpass him or her in skills and freedom; and when brothers and sisters start moving away from home to establish independent lives of their own. This final period is especially painful, since the child with a disability is losing one of his or her caretakers, and depending upon how close the relationship has been, he or she may also be losing a friend and an advocate.

Even before the child with a disability has reached his or her twenty-first birthday, these significant milestones will already have occurred.

Aging-Out

Up until their twenty-first year, through Public Law 94–142, the disabled individual is able to be enrolled in the public school system. Once he reaches twenty-one he is no longer eligible for state-funded education in public schools or Board of Cooperative Education Services (BOCES) locations. As a result, with the aid of his family, he must now seek services through other funding.

The system facing the adult handicapped, however, is dramatically different from the services previously attended. The range of life choices available to people with mental retardation is limited and the sources of rewarding experiences meager. On the level of programming, while in the public school system, the child with a disability experienced services that were rich and offered more variety. But during the aging-out process many individuals will most likely receive services of lesser intensity.

For example, a student who is used to a classroom of six or twelve other students and one or two — or even three — teachers is frequently put into a day treatment program where there are up to twenty individuals per room. Furthermore, the staff in the day treatment program often do not have the same background as special education teachers in the public schools who have master's degrees; typically, program therapists at day treatment programs have at least a high school degree, and although they may have a richness and wealth of experience, they don't have the formal education experiences as staff in the public school system.

The buildings housing the programs available to adults with disabilities further illustrate the contrast of services. As one service provider describes, "This building is an ex-factory; it's been changed into classrooms. One classroom doesn't even have a window."

While parents may have known that services would be scarce once their child reached the age of twenty-one, the reality may not hit them until the time actually comes. As one worker describes, "I think parents believe that their child will be okay as long as he gets adequate services. I think everything fosters that hope and excitement.

"But after twenty-one years, that hope can get somewhat deflated. I'm not saying that that's right; but I really think that happens."

Other workers believe a denial process occurs for a very long time. One worker talks about "a mindset throughout the country that people aren't retarded after the age of eighteen. People may believe that these individuals are cured, or they don't make it. The hope is there, the services are there, and there's also a lot of denial that one's child will grow up to be a mentally retarded adult.

"And then the reality is there. At twenty-one, the services are not as intense as they were prior to that because the school systems have the money. At twenty-one, [individuals find their] services cut unless they are Medicaid eligible. Even then it takes a very long time — it's a very long process — and the same services are not there. And so, parents deal with two realities: (1) my child is

116 | A GUIDE TO MENTAL RETARDATION

now an adult and is still retarded; and (2) we don't get everything we used to in the way of services."

"Kids are also cuter," one worker adds. "People look at kids, and there's always that hope — there's so much hope with children. And when someone becomes an adult, you start to say, 'Is this what it's really going to be like? Is this all there is?' I think that's another reason the hope starts to diminish."

The main reason there are richer services in the education system for the younger handicapped population is primarily due to the bold efforts of parents in the 1950s which, ultimately, initiated Public Law 94–142.

Years ago, many parents were advised to institutionalize children who weren't expected to graduate from school or even live to adulthood; at this time, parents were grateful for whatever they received. However, as the lifestyles and life expectancy of the retarded improved with advancing medical treatment, and as attitudes changed about disabilities, parent's expectations grew. Angry and tired of the lack of specialized programming for their children, parents finally sought the support and funding of their community leaders.

Many of these parents continued their involvement while their children were still in schools through the 1980s. However, after these parents had put so much work into the system, and were getting on in years, it was difficult for them to muster the energy necessary to lobby for further legislative action. One father, recalling the hundreds of hours he put into developing one of the original ARCs, expressed regret that he did not have enough energy to put into continued advocacy for services.

One worker describes the different generations of parents involved in their agency from the beginning. "The parents [at the parents' meetings] are the old timers — the honorary members. They are very supportive of this agency and what it is doing.

"We also have parents who are new to the agency who have these incredible expectations of what we could provide for their child. They are the ones who are saying, 'You don't understand.' "

Another worker talks about dealing with demanding parents: "Sometimes when agencies interact with some parents, they find that there's a certain percentage of parents out there who will be very demanding in terms of the services they expect for their child.

"I think as human beings we sometimes are frustrated by what we have to deal with in our lives, and sometimes this frustration will come out in the face of a direct care worker or clinician. With the parents very disgruntled and wanting more to be done, I think we, as caregivers, need to recognize and be able to address this.

"Also what can happen, what has happened, a parent will come in, I will be sitting there with the parent and the child, and the parent will have expected more to have been accomplished with their son or daughter, and they will react in a way that is demanding — not only to the worker, but also to the child who is sitting there hearing.

"What I'm saying, in general, is that parents have a tremendous burden; they want to see the best accomplished, and occasionally don't have a reasonable perspective."

Yet what we are seeing is that "the commitment found in the parent movement which brought about appropriate public school education for all children with handicaps [needs] to advocate for meaningful employment services." However, there exist only small interest groups who have looked into the attitudes of parents with disabled children or adults toward adult vocational services (Hill, Seyfarth, Banks, Wehman, and Orelove 1987).

"Like anything else, an agency can drift," expresses one worker. "Families may start to take the agency for granted because they weren't the ones who actually did the work to form it. What we need is a revival in the involvement of parents. I think that would be good."

Preparations for Adulthood

Under law, New York schools must begin preparation for adult needs four to six years before a child with a disability turns twenty-one. The process begins when the child is sixteen, where local districts must notify the state education department that a student is aging-out. Parents, as well, are to be informed by the

118 | A GUIDE TO MENTAL RETARDATION

district of the approaching date at which a student will no longer be eligible for state education (Sturgis, *Poughkeepsie Journal*).

School-Based Programs

For youths with all levels of retardation, high school work study programs develop vocational preparation. In this program — running through the student's tenth, eleventh, and twelfth grade — the student spends approximately half of his day in the formal classroom setting, while the other half is spent in vocational instruction. While in the work study program, he receives instruction in learning about jobs that exist in the community, receives assistance to discover personal capabilities and job interests, receives help to develop a wide range of job skills in his area of interest, is exposed to a variety of actual on-the-job experiences under the supervision of the special education facility, and finally helped to find a permanent job.

Sheltered workshops are another option during the high school years. They offer an assortment of job experiences to teach vocational skills and appropriate behaviors to mild, moderate, and severely retarded individuals using simulated work settings. Some are transitional, training clients for eventual competitive employment, placing a strong emphasis on production; while others are long-term or "extended," providing training to individuals who are likely to continue in a particular setting beyond their school years.

Entering the Community

Transitional Issues

For the individual with mental retardation it can be very frustrating, and even devastating, to have school-to-postschool transition disrupted by waiting lists, limited options, and poor coordination of services.

While the transition process presents many roadblocks, opinions about the effectiveness of coordination between schools and adult service agencies vary, even among active contributors to transitional programming (Clark and Knowlton 1987). One such contributor describes an optimistic view, where "there are numerous demonstrations of successful collaboration efforts throughout the country" (Hasazi in Clark et al. 1987).

Another contributor expresses that it might be unrealistic to expect effective coordination, adding that "even when interest in coordination did exist, teachers and administrators had very different perceptions concerning who, if anyone, was responsible for such coordination" (Halpern in Clark et al. 1987). Ideally, of course, professionals work together, share information, and respect each other's roles and expertise. But unfortunately, this may only rarely be the case.

What makes for effective coordination? First, there needs to be frequent communication, trust, and reciprocal understanding of responsibilities between key agency representatives, parents, and advocacy groups; and second, coordination and agreements to share resources are done best at the local level. But in addition to having excellent state inter-agency agreements, we need to keep in mind that real change occurs locally.

Regardless of the current state of effective transition, the attitudes held by parents and caretakers is the strongest force behind any change for a successful outcome. "How well the youngsters make their way depends upon parental expectations and initiative, the availability of suitable jobs and services, the ability to overcome community biases, and luck," one advocate states (*Poughkeepsie Journal*).

Often, families do not receive assistance from an agency at all. "The only way we know people are out there," one worker reports, "is if they have contacted us at some point, or social services contacted us, or the child was in the school at some point and maybe they pulled out and went to BOCES or something and now they're coming back."

"But for a lot of families, the agency has nothing to offer unless they are enrolled in our program. If it's a natural family and they simply want to find out about services, but they don't want to come into the day program, there is not much that we can offer them, except maybe linking them up with other facilities."

Finding a Residential Setting

Finding an appropriate living situation — for example, a group home — is often not so much picking a group home from many alternatives, but finding a home that is available. In many com-

120 | A GUIDE TO MENTAL RETARDATION

munities there are very long waiting lists, up to several years, for a good group home because space is tight.

Many services provided for families have limitations. "We try to educate these families that there may be a five-year waiting period to get into a residence," tells one worker. "Parents should not wait until the last minute when a crisis occurs; for example, when one of the family members has passed on.

"For example, take a mentally retarded adult who is fifty years old, who has lived at home all his life, and whose parents are in their eighties. If a crisis suddenly occurs and the parents can no longer take care of this person what will happen? What usually takes place is that the individual becomes a ward of the state, or he or she goes to a state center. Therefore, parents need to be told to prepare for the eventual separation that's involved, and that it is good for their child — who is really an adult — to be on a waiting list *now*."

Another worker tells of her involvement in parents' groups and transitional committees: "I was asked to be involved with the parents' group. We organized a parents' night, four times a year, to bring parents in to talk about the agency, what we have to offer, and to ask what they want. We asked them if they were getting the services they wanted; if not, what did they need? We asked how they saw the future of the agency, and what we could do for them? We also try to educate parents on how to become involved with their adult children's life.

"I am also involved in a residential transition committee. We invite parents who have a mentally retarded child or adult to come to the meeting to learn about the agency and our resources.

"We try to urge them to think about the future. Right now it might be best for their child to be at home; but ten years from now they may need to make a transition. If they don't start planning for it now, there may be problems.

"Even if they keep the child at home, we teach them what resources are available."

Social Skills vs. Specific Occupational Skills

When preparing the person with a handicap for the adult world, the focus tends to be on teaching them skills specific to the job.

Transition into Adulthood | 121

While this may work in some settings, the need to enhance social skills is also important.

Researchers found that social bonds with nondisabled people can be critical to the functioning of individuals with mental retardation in integrated work environments. Studies are finding that lack of appropriate social skills often plays a bigger part than poor work skills when individuals with severe intellectual disabilities lose their jobs.

Should job coaches and/or trained advocates be used for training in community living skills and personal social skills? Job coaches and trained advocates provide technical assistance in vocational areas to people with severe intellectual disabilities, but these individuals need help with social skills too if they are to learn to utilize the assistance and support of nondisabled others throughout their lives.

Yet advocates also find that the fewer professionals involved in a person's life, the better. So it is vitally important to facilitate and enhance social bonds between people with severe intellectual disabilities and others who are not disabled — preferably others who are not paid to be with them.

Sometimes individuals with disabilities may not want to pursue employment. One state agency has a policy on transitional programming stating that individuals leaving the school system need to obtain jobs, and that that promotes community integration. But some people with disabilities may not choose to work for good reasons, and furthermore, may choose to spend most of their time in the company of other people with disabilities.

The reactions to this issue are many. "It may depend upon what is best for that individual and who makes the judgment call," one worker comments. "If the parents are the legal guardians, they have the right to make the decision for their child. However, the way the system is right now they won't get any services."

Other persons have argued that a person, to be normalized, may have to face the same consequences that all people have to face if unemployed. "Our people have not been trained to make choices," another worker presents. "Most people who are mentally retarded have been taken care of for all of their lives.

"If they're at home, in an institution, in a residence, they are told, 'This is what you're going to do. This is how you do it.' They've never been taught what it is to make a choice. They've

122 | A GUIDE TO MENTAL RETARDATION

never been asked, 'Do you want to work, or do you want to stay home?'

"Instead it's, 'You're getting up, you're going to day treatment Monday through Friday from 9:00 to 4:00,' or 'You're going to work, and on Saturday and Sunday this is what we're going to do.' So there's a whole educational process needed to help people understand the consequences of their decisions. The mentally retarded adult has not been given that opportunity. It is only a recent awakening."

Transition Needs for the Adult with Mild Disabilities

There exists a distinction in the transition needs and employment patterns between adults with severe retardation and those who are mildly retarded (Neubert, Tilson, and Ianacone 1989). While the vocational training, employment, and long-term follow-up needs of persons with severe disabilities receive federal and state attention, the needs of persons with mild disabilities — who outnumber the population of severely retarded by a ratio of 10 to 1 — have not been as evident.

It is the common assumption in delivery of services that persons with mild disabilities are able to move from school to work with greater ease than those with severe disabilities (Rushch and Phelps 1987 in Neubert et al. 1989). Furthermore, it is assumed that a majority of individuals with mild retardation need only time-limited services, such as assistance from a work-study coordinator or vocational rehabilitation counselor (Will 1984 in Neubert et al. 1989).

But current research provides little support for these assumptions. One group of researchers (Neubert et al. 1989) suggests that transition should encompass more than the movement from school to a particular job. Furthermore, the success of transition or employment outcomes should consider economic self-sufficiency, not just the individual's ability to access an initial job. Since job changes are a natural part of the employment process, continued support is necessary to accomplish job changes and advancement.

Transition into Adulthood | 123

Career Opportunities for Moderately to Profoundly Retarded Adults

Another observable difference between adults who are mildly retarded and those who have moderate to profound retardation is behavior. As a result, the career opportunities for the groups will vary.

The behavior of adults with mild retardation — approximately 80% of the population labeled retarded — only minimally reduces their career options; the vast majority of them will be capable of independent living as adults, and many will no longer be labeled or recognized as mentally retarded after they leave school (Patton, Payne, and Beirne-Smith 1986).

"Persons with mild retardation go into supported work situations or even regular jobs," one worker reports. "We have people that work in the kitchen at [many community placements]. Some people are doing dishes, some are chambermaids making the beds — they're doing blue-collar work. There are some working at McDonald's running the cash registers and getting the orders out."

On the other hand, persons with moderate to severe retardation — approximately 20% of the population of mentally retarded people — exhibit patterns of behavior that disrupt their learning and interaction with others so much that their career options are sharply limited. As adults, they will frequently be dependent upon support from others in order to function within the community (Patton et al. 1986).

"The more severe the mental retardation is," one worker reports, "the lower the cognitive level. We have people with cognitive levels of a two-year-old. There are not many jobs that a two-year-old would be capable of doing."

Problems with Adjustment

Mentally retarded persons have varying degrees of success in adjusting to life following school. In some cases, however, when the adult handicapped is admitted to a new program — usually settings where the individual requires more supervision — one

124 | A GUIDE TO MENTAL RETARDATION

unfortunate thing that occurs is that some individuals may react with behavioral problems. In many cases, this is not due to problems within themselves or their family, but rather to the disappearance of the supportive network that existed during their school years.

One mother describes her situation: "Craig does not adjust well to change. . . . He had a very hard adjustment to the day treatment program. I think it was difficult for Craig because he was used to having other boys in his class who, although they were all retarded like Craig, had very normal behavior. They talked and went to the cafeteria with the other kids. He was exposed to the regular student population in the high school. Now he is exposed to all retarded people, with a majority of them more retarded than he is." She adds, "Craig is very aware that he is now with all of these retarded people. . . . Some of their behavior is different, and I think it bothers Craig to realize that this is where he is."

An educational coordinator describes the situation for one individual: "Ben really did not have a chance to develop a lot of internal controls because he was not left to his own devices for long periods of time. Public school was so structured an environment. There was always someone around him and always someone helping him. Ben gets into a day treatment setting where, yes, there is work provided, but one person is taking care of eight to ten clients and staff need to move over to somebody else for awhile. That's when Ben really has problems. . . . It's very hard for him."

As a master's level psychologist, a significant part of the job is addressing behavioral problems such as these. It often becomes frustrating for the staff when assisting the retarded adult to work through a behavioral outburst — frustrating not only because of the behavioral outburst itself and its threat to the personal safety of those involved, but knowing that the feelings behind these behaviors are legitimate in the mind of the person. At times, it seems as if the adult service agency, at some level, is expecting the retarded individual, who recently has aged out from a richer environment, to adapt to, and be satisfied with, his or her new — yet limited — surroundings, when he or she has the need for a more supportive service.

Other families are fortunate enough not to experience the full impact of the change in the teacher/client ratio. One mother

Transition into Adulthood | 125

describes the support she and her daughter received: "The staff was caring and attentive. A lot of my questions were answered. I felt that Sarah's future was in good hands."

Future Trends in Transition Programming

Various opinions exist concerning the emerging trends in the field of transitional programming (Clark and Knowlton 1987). They are as follows:

— "More and more parents and advocates are going to insist on real employment before students leave school, as prevocational, simulated, or other pretend types of work fall increasingly into disfavor with many school systems" (Wehman in Clark et al. 1987).

— "The eligibility requirements for vocational rehabilitation services are beginning to blur . . . as more and more students, previously thought to be ineligible because of functioning level, are exhibiting vocational competence" (Wehman in Clark et al. 1987).

— "More students are moving into better paying manufacturing positions and are less concentrated in the entry-level service positions such as dishwashers or potscrubbers" (Wehman in Clark et al. 1987).

— Students with handicaps will be allowed "to build a work history prior to graduation" which will "increase their prospects for employment following high school" (Hasazi in Clark et al. 1987).

— "Unlike school, adult services are not guaranteed." Therefore, "parents have become more aware of the vulnerability of their children and are more involved in lifelong planning" (Brown in Clark et al. 1987).

— Professionals will be looking "at the requirements of adulthood and then devote the last ten years of education to teaching students to behave and function as effectively as possible in integrated environments and activities," rather than "spending the adolescent years trying to take students with disabilities through normal infant development stages and phases" (Brown in Clark et al. 1987).

— Rather than preparing people with disabilities to spend the years from age twenty-one to seventy in segregated activity centers

126 | A GUIDE TO MENTAL RETARDATION

or sheltered workshops, "more adult service agencies are providing integrated options, and more professionals have the values, skills, and experiences necessary to provide quality services" (Brown in Clark et al. 1987).

Special Training

Persons with mental retardation who are considered job-ready and employable often have difficulty creating a favorable impression with potential employers due to social skills deficits in the job interview setting. A number of studies have demonstrated that social skills training can improve the self-presentation and social appearance of applicants with mental retardation (Kelly and Christoff 1985).

Successful interventions are based upon a "package" of behavioral training techniques (Kelly 1982 in Kelly and Christoff 1985). These include instructions and coaching on basic interview skills; modeling to demonstrate appropriate behavior; opportunities to practice or role-play in simulated job interviews; and feedback, reinforcement, and refinement of these skills. Since the aim of intervention is to change a trainee's behavior in the "real world," it is important to provide training of sufficient intensity to teach skills that will be maintained (Kelly and Christoff 1985). Group interventions which provide evidence that skills are generalized to realistic settings typically require sixteen to twenty-four sessions.

Assertiveness Training

Research suggests that persons with mental retardation tend to have personality characteristics which lead to nonassertive behavior (Bregman 1985). It has been demonstrated, however, that adults with mental retardation are capable of learning to express themselves assertively and in a proper manner (Bregman 1984 in Bregman 1985); and because the experiences related to assertive behavior feel good and are self-rewarding, these skills can be learned quickly.

The Elwyn Institute has developed a helpful assertiveness training program designed specifically for the population of

Transition into Adulthood | 127

persons with retardation (illustrated in Bregman 1985). The program is divided into six sessions and is best orchestrated in a group setting.

The first session focuses on the use of appropriate affect and the expression of feelings. This is done through identifying and explaining the emotion depicted in various pictures and by acting out the appropriate emotion relating to situations, such as "your boss has given you a compliment about your work."

Expressing needs and desires is the focus of the second session. In the time that I have worked with adults with mental retardation, this is one area that I have found to be in need of assistance. When the disabled person, or anyone for that matter, has difficulty expressing needs, it can lead to frustration and dissatisfaction. Therefore, this session involves ways of letting others know how you feel, what you want, and what you need, for such area as requesting help for a medical problem, asking for a raise, and so on.

The third session helps with appropriate expressions of anger. Through role-play, individuals are asked to respond to different situations; for example, "children are snickering at you and calling you names at a store. What would you do?" By dealing with the issue of anger, the individual is able to realize that everyone feels anger and that the way anger is expressed has to do with what one has learned. The individual soon discovers that previous inappropriate behavior can be modified.

Learning how to say no appropriately is the focus of the fourth session. Learning this skill can aid a person with a disability to deal with pushy salespersons and drug pushers, and to stand up to unreasonable demands made by those requesting that he or she sign his or her name without knowing the reason.

Final sessions help the person express his or her opinions, while respecting the opinions of others, and assert himself or herself to authority figures, as many adults with retardation are often afraid to speak up for fear of saying or doing the wrong thing and getting into trouble.

Self-Management Training

Most behavior therapies aimed toward persons with mental retardation involve modifications to the individual's setting through

128 | A GUIDE TO MENTAL RETARDATION

the aid of counselors, teachers, aids, and parents. While effective, there is a disadvantage to relying too much on these external sources, limited maintenance, and generalization of learned appropriate behaviors. Some have concerns that the individual has limited involvement in the training process.

Self-management training, therefore, is designed to teach skills that can be used in a deliberate manner to change one's own behavior, including skills in self-monitoring, self-evaluation, implementing one's own consequences, and self-instruction.

Results of various research (illustrated in Cole and Gardner 1984) demonstrate that individuals with mental retardation, ranging from mild to profound, and from children to adults, can learn various skills of self-management, and these procedures are at least as effective as similar externally managed methods in aiding positive behavior change. Examples of positive behavior changes include an increase in work productivity, a reduction in socially undesirable behaviors, a decrease in disruptive behavior, and so on (Cole and Gardner 1984).

Working with Families

A normal process of separation from home cannot occur in families where there is a retarded individual. No matter how independent and self-sufficient a retarded person becomes, it simply is not the same as having a child who can go out, find a good job, get married, and return home or live nearby as a self-sufficient adult in the community. Because of this, many parents suffer conflict.

"If one of my children were retarded," one worker empathized, "and I realized that they would never be able to survive without a support system around them — they were not going to go out, get married, and have children — that's a very heavy guilt trip to put on oneself. It's very hard to deal with dimmed dreams and aspirations that a parent would have wanted for their child."

"Parents also may feel that no one can ever replace mom and dad," another worker adds. "It's hard to let go."

"A lot of times when the [clients move] into a residence, they are made responsible for their own room, responsible for their laundry, responsible to help do the cooking and make their own lunch.

"While the adult had been living at home, most families still look at their offspring as children. The family did the laundry, the family made the lunches; they take total care of them and, unfortunately, never let the retarded person grow up.

"There have been conflicts between parents and agencies, where parents are angry that the agency staff is making their child perform all of these duties; it's hard for them to understand that it is good and that it is all right. That letting go of their forty-year-old adult is good."

Another area of conflict often occurs between families and junior staff members. Some young staff members, in enthusiasm for their new jobs, see their role as providing advice for parents. This contrasts seasoned therapists, who see their role as helping families clarify all issues and then come to an informed decision. In the latter case, the therapist realizes that it is the family's decision of what to do. Sometimes, junior staff members see their role as the decision-makers, or the agency's role as the decision-maker, and this causes friction if not outright hostility between these staff members, the agency, and parents.

"There may be more problems with parents of persons in the supportive work. With a lot of supportive work and higher functioning individuals, the families are still very much involved. These people have never really been in institutions; they've been at home all of their lives. I do know that there have been times when parents feel that the residential care is inadequate, and they want more freedom for their child."

How can they remain involved and helpful with their adult children and allow enough independence for healthy development to occur? This is a troubling question for every parent. Some parents try to resolve this issue by keeping their adult child at home. This may work out very well if there is an extended family with many friends around.

Sometimes, a widowed husband or wife will attempt to keep an adult child at home. In these situations there can be problems when the adult child does not have the level of stimulation and social contacts that might happen at a placement.

While conflicts and dissatisfaction do occur, most parents are generally pleased with the services they receive. As one worker describes, "Basically, I don't think this agency has many problems with families. There are people who come in to help bake cookies

130 | A GUIDE TO MENTAL RETARDATION

for our clients. A great portion of parents are grateful for the services we provide."

Options in the Community

"We are really struggling to understand where exactly adults with mental retardation fit into our culture. Not forcing them in, but where do they *fit* in?

"There are different ways to look at the history, but you are still left with the same question: Where do they fit in? In [our] state, they're saying, 'Yeah, fit them into supportive work.' Meanwhile, our economy is not doing very well."

One administrator has seen this situation: "There are 380,000 unemployed people in [this one] state alone who are not mentally retarded. And then you're saying, 'Let's put our people into supportive work and put them out into the community,' but it's hard to compete.

"The reality is, if there are two people applying for a job, and one is a husband trying to support a family and the other is a mentally retarded adult who is provided with room and board, clothing, and everything else, the decision will obviously favor the family man in need of money."

According to one research group: "The quality of life for each person with mental retardation depends, in part, upon the availability of appropriate community resources. Only through having a variety of experiences and opportunities to develop and assume responsibilities does the individual have the chance to function as close to 'normalization' as he or she can" (Patton et al. 1986).

That variety of experiences and opportunities implies options for the mentally retarded in the areas of employment, housing, and leisure. And work is just as significant for the person with mental retardation as it is for anyone. Fortunately, social changes and changes in public policy have allowed more people with disabilities to participate in the work force and share the benefits of gainful employment.

Individuals with severe retardation, once thought to possess little potential for gainful employment, are now demonstrating the ability to perform complex work tasks when provided with appropriate and systematic training (Bellamy 1979 in Patton et al.

1986). Furthermore, the Rehabilitations Act of 1983 has mandated that existing vocational programs and resources include persons with handicaps (Patton et al. 1986).

Day Treatment Programming

Day treatment programs provide daytime activities for persons with more severe retardation who require a higher level of structure, supervision, and support. This population is older than school age and considered to be too handicapped to maintain the levels of production necessary within workshop settings. However, some persons may move on to these settings if, after receiving adequate training, they demonstrate maintenance of their newly acquired skills. One worker describes one such situation: "There are people who have graduated from day treatment to sheltered work, and they are very happy. They are now getting a check every two weeks."

Another version of day treatment programming includes being in a sheltered workshop for part of the day. One program has set up a separate program between the day treatment and sheltered workshop, a six-month transitional program which provides more intensive work skills training for individuals with a high potential for advancement to the workshop.

Day treatment centers provide training in prevocational and vocational skills; this may include simple assembly tasks such as sorting markers or nuts and bolts. However, employability is not the main focus; the program stresses increased self-sufficiency through a greater emphasis on teaching daily living skills such as travel, safety, grooming, and communication.

Increasing recreation and socialization are also included, as well as the opportunity for work and pay. At one day treatment location, program therapists put great efforts into obtaining realistic play money and a cash register with which to simulate spending at an in-house store.

Clients may be in a classroom setting with up to twenty peers and two staff. However, for clients in need of a more intensive arrangement due to special behavioral, intellectual, or medical needs, there may be six to eight peers per room for every two staff. For example, one individual experienced overwhelming levels of anxiety and paced back and forth in the classroom. When she wasn't getting the attention she needed, she would occasion-

132 | A GUIDE TO MENTAL RETARDATION

ally hit her peers. It was difficult to intervene with her in the larger classroom, and so the smaller, more structured setting was considered more able to meet her needs.

Sheltered Workshops

Sheltered workshops offer an assortment of job experiences to train vocational skills and necessary work habits with the goal of eventually obtaining salaried employment. The workshop may serve persons with mild, moderate, and severe retardation, and often individuals with other handicapping conditions.

A sheltered workshop may be classified in three different ways (Patton et al. 1986): (1) Transitional workshops concentrate on the development of vocational skills, placing a strong emphasis on production, to help the disabled worker — mainly persons with mild retardation — to eventually gain employment in the community; (2) Extended or "long-term" workshops provide long-term employment to individuals — usually in the moderate, severe, and profound range of retardation — who cannot secure employment at competitive industries and will remain dependent on the workshop for future employment; and (3) Comprehensive workshops are the most common — they include both transitional and extended services.

Within these settings, clients usually work on contractual jobs — usually of short duration, where most tasks are broken down into small steps which are set up in assembly-line fashion; for example, one female worker describes how she puts lipstick containers together and then boxes them. Nonvocational services are also frequently provided to assist adults in personal and social adjustment, including the ability to handle money, self-care, and recreation.

Sheltered workshops have been attempting to meet the needs of persons with more severe retardation, but several criticisms have been cited (Schalock 1983). First, persons with handicaps, in general, often lack movement from the workshop into competitive work sites; liaisons between sheltered workshops and private business or industry are generally limited to lacking. Furthermore, most contracts received from participating local industries provide workers only menial, monotonous tasks, "which limit the possibility for maximizing the potential of all clients in the workshop" (Patton et al. 1986).

Some workers question the future of sheltered work, based upon current financial strains. "This is something that is receiving less funding now," one worker explains. "Sheltered work is losing favor because it is not completely out in the community."

The problem becomes apparent when contracting work to be done in the workshops. "The agency has employed people to go out and beat the bushes and say, 'Get us this contract; Give us this work.' And in a shrinking economy, the people at the bottom of the totem pole are the first ones to feel the effect."

Transitional Employment

Between the sheltered workshop and competitive employment, there may be a transitional phase which allows clients the opportunity to generalize the skills learned within the sheltered workshop. Transitional employment allows for decreasing supervision and increasing personal autonomy as well as integration through preparation and control of the work environment.

Another approach involves the use of job coaches. After a suitable place of employment has been found for a client, a job coach will accompany the client to the job site and provide any assistance the worker may need in adapting to the new environment. This service is provided as long as the job coach is needed, during which time the service is faded out to once a week or once a month, depending upon the individual.

Competitive Employment

In competitive placements, individuals with retardation are employed in regular jobs in the community and are paid for their work. These jobs are usually unskilled or semiskilled labor; for example, some individuals obtain jobs doing janitorial work, while others may bag groceries at local supermarkets.

One individual tells of the many different job experiences he has had: "Right now I'm doing recycling . . . collecting plastic bottles, newspapers, and cans. Before, I was washing dishes at a hotel, and before that, I worked at the bowling alley sweeping floors." Other individuals may be self-employed and hire themselves out as yardworkers or housekeepers. Most persons with retardation who find jobs in competitive employment are mildly retarded; however, there are examples of persons with severe

134 | A GUIDE TO MENTAL RETARDATION

handicaps working as cafeteria and fountain attendants, baker's helpers and duplicating machine operators (Cook et al. 1977 in Patton et al. 1986).

Employment Issues

"Two of the biggest things that control where people work, besides their intelligence level, is their behavior and their ability to attend to tasks," one worker explains. "There are a number of people in the day treatment program that have the ability to work in a workshop, or even in supportive work; but their behavior is not adequate — they have no self-control, or their attention span is very, very short." As a result, many of these people need to remain in the more supportive, yet less challenging, setting.

At times, a situation like this seems like a Catch-22. If the individual is high-functioning enough to work independently, but because of his or her behavior he or she needs to be in a more supervised situation, it unfortunately supplies less stimulating work or activities, and that boredom may feed a behavioral fire since the individual may need more challenging work.

"An example," one worker illustrates," is an individual with a fairly high intelligence who was in a sheltered workshop. However, she would kick and scream that she didn't want to go to work.

"Finally, the psychologist came to talk with her and found out that she hated coming to the sheltered workshop. What she wanted to do was sweep the floors in a church; she wanted to do porter maintenance at a church right down the street from where she lived. It was investigated, we talked with the pastor, and that is what she is doing today. She has not had a behavior problem since. She simply didn't like her job, and didn't want to get up every morning to go to what she considered a horrible place.

The environment has changed, not the individual. It's sad that we don't always have the staffing or the ability necessary to do this all of the time."

A coworker relates his own experiences with limited job opportunities: "I know for myself — I've gone through many different jobs in my life — at one point I worked in a factory. I hated it. I absolutely hated it. If I was put into a situation where that was the only job I could do, who knows what my behaviors would be and where I would be today. Not everyone is geared to work in a factory."

Ideally the efforts made to assist persons with developmental disabilities in the working environment — the level of structure needs depends upon their level of functioning — includes attempts to capitalize on the strengths they have — both hidden and apparent — to create as independent a lifestyle as possible.

The importance of work cannot be argued; the potential gains in one's self-esteem are undoubtedly important. Even for persons with disabilities, "competitive employment . . . enhances feelings of self-worth and efficacy and increases the normalization of these people, both in self-perception and the perception of society" (Scott and Sarkees 1982 in Schloss, Wolf, and Schloss 1987).

Increased financial well-being is often assumed to be another benefit of employment for persons with disabilities. However, financial problems may arise for persons with disabilities to work, since "income gained from employment may not offset the withdrawal of federal support." In fact, it has been made apparent that current state and federal programs, in general, do not provide many incentives for handicapped adults to enter the work force. For example, researchers found the net income to be practically the same for individuals working part-time and those working full-time (Schloss et al. 1987).

"In sheltered workshops, there are time studies," explains one agency supervisor, clarifying the system used at her place of employment. "The person's abilities are compared with a 'normal' person's in terms of how much work they can do. The federal government checks the money on an annual basis. They come in to make sure the agency is paying the client the appropriate wage. The worker is getting paid for what they do by the same production/payment ratio as the general population."

The satisfaction received from a job comes, in part, from the conditions in which one works. This includes the safety and appealing nature of the environment, relationships with coworkers, quality of supervision, and hours of work. When any one of these areas is not to our satisfaction, we have the means to seek out improvements.

Individuals with mental retardation do not have the full range of experience or cognitive abilities to evaluate the conditions of their workplace. They may feel they do not have much of a choice in the type of setting in which they work.

One woman with relatively mild retardation, when asked about her feelings as to her placement, even replied, "Do I have a

136 | A GUIDE TO MENTAL RETARDATION

choice?" revealing the possible feelings of persons with retardation in general who, because of political reasons or desires of agencies, caretakers, etc., have basically learned not to participate in placement decisions.

Work environments for the individual with retardation do not always provide for adequate job satisfaction. For example, sheltered workshops are designed on the assumption that individuals with retardation can work only on simple tasks, and that such persons have virtually no growth needs and their ability to perform somewhat complicated tasks is limited. However, some believe that the simple, routine jobs that are provided at a sheltered workshop lead to boredom and low productivity (Shapira, Cnaan, and Cnaan 1985).

One worker provides a different perspective on job satisfaction for persons with mental retardation: "I think it depends upon the individual. One thing we have to realize is that there is a different mindset in a person with a different intelligence level. There is nothing bad about that.

"You could have a genius who could be totally bored doing my job, and yet I enjoy my job. You could have a person who is mentally retarded sweeping floors and enjoying it; they are getting a charge out of the way the dirt is being moved in a certain direction, or the shape of the floor — things we would not normally focus on. For them, it may be totally fulfilling.

"I think that one of our problems is that a lot of our sheltered work is factory-type work, and always will be. Some people like factory work, and some don't. If we could come up with alternative sheltered work besides just factory work, that would be good.

"Here in the northeast there's not a lot of farm work. There is a big difference between someone who is mentally retarded living in New York City and someone living in Oklahoma. In our area clients haven't been exposed to many opportunities.

"The key to understanding is to find out what they are enjoying or not enjoying and what they have to say about it."

For a person with mental retardation — usually those functioning below the level of mild retardation — it may be unreasonable to expect them to advocate for an adequate working environment. Sometimes, such concerns are left to parents who unfortunately may not have accurate information about their child's working environment and, this may result in low expectations of a job placement.

While interviewing parents of persons with moderate retardation, researchers found that most of these parents were satisfied with the current program placements for their adult children (Hill, Seyfarth, Banks, and Orelove 1987).

One study concludes that parents' attitudes may be shaped by what they see in the community; therefore, "as more and more local programs provide better paying, integrated employment alternatives and clients are successful in those jobs, parents will begin to change their expectations for the types of services they desire" (Hill et al. 1987).

Residential Placement

A person's transition into the work force is not the only consideration in aging-out. There eventually comes the time when the question of leaving home arises — whether in the individual himself or in the parents.

The following are general descriptions of community living arrangements found in many parts of the country.

Intermediate Care Facilities (ICF-MR)

Located in the community, Intermediate Care Facilities for persons with mental retardation provide twenty-four-hour care to its population; this includes nursing, medical support, training, and therapeutic support (Patton et al. 1986). This setting provides an intensive level of supervision, and independent adaptive functioning is limited significantly.

Community Residences

Community residences, or group homes, are the most common community living arrangement (Patton et al. 1986). Within these homes, adults receive support and supervision from counselors. Some residences are transitional in focus, preparing adults to move to more independent situations, while others may serve as long-term living arrangements. A greater level of independence and self-care is expected of individuals who live in community residences in comparison to those who live in an ICF program.

138 | A GUIDE TO MENTAL RETARDATION

Group homes are typically small. They may have ten or fewer adult residents — usually mildly or moderately retarded — two staff members, and a relief staff (Patton et al. 1986). Adults in these homes are frequently involved in a day activity or are employed.

Group homes may also be larger, holding from eleven to twenty, twenty-one to forty, or forty-one to eighty residents. These larger group homes offer a more specialized, professional staff and usually serve persons who are older and more handicapped. Since there is a lower staff-to-client ratio, they tend to be more restrictive and provide fewer opportunities for resident autonomy or involvement in decision-making (Patton et al. 1986).

Protective Settings

Other settings which offer support to individuals with mental retardation include family care and sheltered communities. In family care settings, the person with mental retardation is integrated into the home of a family that has been recruited from the community.

In their ideal form, these homes create a warm, family atmosphere that provides adults with a normalized life within the community (Stoneman and Crapps 1988), although there may be some variability as to how well these homes create this atmosphere.

People who offer their services as family care providers, as research in the field shows, are unique individuals themselves. The majority of family care providers are middle-aged or older; most are married with children. Single home providers are usually widows; many have adult children who have left home (Willer and Intagliata 1984 in Stoneman and Crapps 1988). The education and income levels of family care providers tend to be below the national average (Intagliata, Crosby, and Nelder 1981 in Stoneman and Crapps 1988). In addition, it is not uncommon for family care providers to have worked with persons with mental retardation or for the provider to have a family member with a handicapping condition (Justice, Bradley, and O'Connor 1971 in Stoneman and Crapps 1988).

Sheltered communities, on the other hand, are typically located outside the immediate community. Some of these settings attempt to insulate individuals with disabilities from a public that is viewed as unable or unlikely to accept handicapped adults (Patton et al. 1986).

Community Training Programs

Workshop dormitories have been developed in some areas as boarding school-type models for individuals working in sheltered workshops and attending a vocational training arm of the workshop (Patton et al. 1986). These training programs and dormitories are generally transitional in nature.

Similar training models also exist on the grounds of some institutions, and offer preparation programs if and when the adults are deinstitutionalized (Patton et al. 1986).

Supervised Apartments

Apartment programs represent the least restrictive environment alternatives within the community residential programming and provide a setting for living and learning the skills necessary for community living and integration (Patton et al. 1986).

Residents in these programs are usually less severely handicapped and have better personal and social adjustment skills. Most are employed competitively or at workshops (Patton et al. 1986).

The degree of supervision, support, and training provided to the adult depends upon the individual's particular needs. Some may require support with money, cooking, and/or household skills, while others may demand services only at times of crisis (Patton et al. 1986).

One supervised apartment arrangement may involve a non-disabled individual sharing an apartment, or even a home, with one or more persons with mental retardation, receiving support and assistance on a periodic basis from a nonresident staff person.

Specialized Communities

While most programs for adults with mental retardation focus on molding or training the individual to function within the society, there exist several select programs throughout the world that emphasize an alternative philosophy, where the environment is altered to accommodate the individual. Most of these programs create

140 | A GUIDE TO MENTAL RETARDATION

discrete societies where persons with mental retardation may live "sheltered from the rejection and failures too often experienced in society" (Patton et al. 1986).

The founders of such programs believe that, in this type of protective environment, persons with mental retardation "can achieve a feeling of belonging, develop their own social connections, and enjoy useful, productive lives." Furthermore, "because they are self-contained and ideally self-sufficient communities, one could argue that these programs are normal in the same way that an ethnic community could be a normal, though different, segment of the larger community" (Patton et al. 1986).

"There are places which have been successful around our area," notes Dan Forte. "There's a farm on the other side of the river. There are lots of different houses on the farm, and a few individuals with mental retardation living with families in each home. People dedicate their lives to living in community with people who are mentally retarded. They've had some great success with this type of situation."

Some characteristics of these communities may include the following (Patton et al. 1986):

(a) There is no staff-client distinction;

(b) There is an emphasis on established healthy interpersonal relationships and a sense of communal living;

(c) All members of the community share the ownership and profits of labor as equal partners; and

(d) These communities tend to require that each member be able to care for his or her own physical needs and require no medical or custodial care.

Individualized Residential Alternatives (IRA)

Following suit to other states, New York State is currently developing Individual Residential Alternatives. If the person with a disability needs some form of supervised environment, a building can be certified by the state, separate from other waiver services.

These new supervised homes, in essence, will become the "new wave" of Intermediate Care Facilities (ICF) and community residences in the state. "The general thrust of the Individualized Residential Alternatives (IRA)," as one worker describes, "is to provide smaller living environments. The days of eight-, ten-, and twelve-bed homes are over. We will be looking at living environments for people that are much more normalized in size and arrangement."

"Let's say a person is in a community residence (CR)," another worker illustrates, "and their health changed to the point where they weren't able to stay in a CR setting anymore (the support at a CR is different than at an ICF because of staff-client ratio). By today's standards, that person would then have to be switched to an ICF.

"With an IRA, on the other hand, if the person at the CR suddenly needed more services, they could bring more staff into the setting to provide the services. The houses would be built and funded by the needs of the individuals who live there."

Leisure

Like all people, the individual with mental retardation needs recreational activities to provide a change in his or her daily schedule and to prevent boredom. One author states that persons with mental retardation "can advance in health and physical fitness, mobility, language, social skills, and self-esteem through participation in recreational activities" (Patton et al. 1986).

But unfortunately most persons with mental retardation remain outside the mainstream of community life with regard to recreational activities (Patton et al. 1986). The recreational repertoire of these individuals generally consists of passive events such as watching television or movies, listening to records, walking, and looking at magazines.

Many adults who are retarded do not have recreational skills because of limited experience or instruction, slow or uneven physical development, or the lack of friends with whom to learn or play (Patton et al. 1986).

"Many people who have been working in a workshop all of their lives suddenly couldn't handle leisure because there was choice involved," one worker describes. "They just don't have anything they like to do. Their whole life was: get up in the morning, get dressed, eat, go off to work, come home, eat, watch television, go to sleep. They never really had the choice to develop any leisure-type activities. They didn't know what arts-and-crafts were. They didn't know what it was like to go bowling. They

142 | A GUIDE TO MENTAL RETARDATION

didn't know what it was like to go on a boat. They've never done any of these things before."

The program this woman supervises provides exposure to leisure activities. "We are also teaching our clients how to deal with and understand the idea of choice; that it is okay to get up in the morning and think, 'What do I want to do today?' "

"The Medicaid Waiver will have a tremendous effect on the possibilities for activities and leisure. The case manager's role is to ask the client, 'What do you want to do?' And the client can respond, 'I would like to continue going to day treatment two days a week, but I also would like to go to the YMCA, I would like to go join a senior center, I would like to stay at home one day a week and just watch the soap operas or bake cookies.' "

The Decision to Remain at Home

In the past, the general attitude was to exclude persons with mental retardation from society and to isolate them from their families. Today, the current emphasis is on normalization, deinstitutionalization, community integration, and quality of life (Blatt 1987 in Cole and Meyer 1989).

As Benson and Turnbull (1986) later observed, "The movement away from institutionalization and other out-of-home placements for children with severe disabilities has generated a need to assist families in keeping their children at home until they reach adulthood."

Unfortunately, as Cole and Meyer later discovered, services have focused exclusively on out-of-home placements with little focus on approaches to in-home family support that facilitates maintenance in the community. Other researchers observe that children who are living at home and those with more severe disabilities "are less likely to receive services compared to those who live away from their families or have less severe disabilities" (Bjaanes, Butler, and Kelly 1981 in Cole and Meyer 1989).

Providing for the needs of the individual with a disability at home, while encouraging, is not that simple. As one worker in the field describes, "The way matters are today, if you were to keep this person at home and you were totally taking care of this person yourself, you wouldn't be able to supply the things that this person needed — equipment is too expensive. Unless, however, you were economically in need, or the church helped out. It used to be based upon what the family's income was. If the family was 'middle America,' they were not going to get any services for this individual."

"A situation such as this put a real strain on families. 'Do we keep our child at home, where we're not able to do anything?' one parent asked, 'or do we let go of them and put them in the hands of an agency?' "

The Waiver: Part of an Economic Move

Since the advent of the Medicaid Waiver, the door has been opened to provide more services that were previously unattainable. As one worker describes: "Now, with the Medicaid Waiver, the family can apply for Waiver services, regardless of their income. You can get a ramp built to your house, or adaptive equipment for the bathroom."

People apply for Medicaid status, which is an application to a federal program. Then they request equipment they need to keep their child at home; for example, a motorized wheelchair, a ramp, adaptive equipment in the kitchen or the bathroom. Medicaid gives up to $9,000 a year to provide for each individual.

"In reality it is much cheaper for the federal government and the state to give $9,000 for services to an individual to be able to stay home than to place them in an ARC residence or an institution. The Medicaid Waiver is part of an economic move."

What is involved in the decision to place the child in an agency or to keep the child at home? According to various studies (Tausig 1985 in Cole and Meyer 1989), the following reasons were provided when families were interviewed:

(1) the number of children living at home;

(2) resources available to the family to cope with the demands of the child;

(3) the disruption of family relationships;

(4) stressors such as the burden of care;

(5) the ability to access external resources (that is, in-home child care and medical assistance, medical and dental professionals able to work with mentally retarded persons, etc.);

(6) family health problems;

(7) multiple problems within the family;

144 | A GUIDE TO MENTAL RETARDATION

(8) the level of disability and/or frequency of behavior problems.

Families with high levels of internal resources — for example, well-adjusted, high-functioning families with higher incomes — were more apt to report plans for keeping their child at home indefinitely or at least until the age of twenty-one.

Once the decision is made, many factors contribute to the success of keeping the child at home past age twenty-one. According to Seltzer and Krauss (1989), several factors were involved:

(a) the age, marital status, education, and income of the parents;

(b) maternal physical health and life satisfaction;

(c) the level of retardation and whether a child has Down syndrome;

(d) physical health and functional skills of the individual;

(e) parent's ability to cope with stress.

The family's social climate is a better predictor of maternal well-being than formal or informal support. Seltzer et al. (1989) further add that "it appears that the parenting role remains a central part of mother's identity, even into old age."

When asked to name those resources parents felt would contribute most to their ability to maintain their child or adult offspring at home, Cole and Meyer (1989) elicited the following responses:

(a) spousal assistance (which ranked first);

(b) coverage of medical and dental expenses;

(c) evening and weekend in-home child care;

(d) extra funds for help around the house;

(e) professional consultation for behavior problems;

(f) a physician who is knowledgeable about children with severe handicaps;

(g) special transportation to daily activities;

(h) funds for special equipment;

(i) out-of-home respite care facilities; and

(j) access to community recreational programs for their child.

While concerns exist about the services that can be procured from the community while the individual with a developmental disability stays at home, some workers and parents wonder if staying home is the best environment for the individual.

"Depending upon their level of disability," one worker explains, "it may be better for them to move on in their lives, to grow up, and not always be at home with mom and dad."

Respite Care

While not always readily available, respite care is currently a popular and growing concept in service provision. It consists of providing temporary day or night relief services to families caring at home for persons with development disabilities. Since the services enable the disabled person to remain with the family, respite care assures continuity of normal living patterns for the persons involved (Grant and McGrath 1990).

As one worker explains: "Respite care is given to families in need. Say a family wants to go on vacation for two weeks, they would ask for someone to take care of their daughter while they are away. We would then look for respite facilities for the individual. As is the case in some of our residences, if one of our clients is in a crisis situation and the residence or the natural family can't handle the situation, then we would find an alternative placement for the time being."

There are a number of respite models in use. "If it is a state employee," one supervisor reports, "there is a thirty-day respite at a nearby institution. Our agency provides people who are paid to take clients into their homes. There are people who sign up to be respite providers. They get paid so much an hour to take these people into their home for a weekend, several weeks, or over vacations. One woman offered to take an individual from the natural family for respite every weekend."

Based upon a study done by Grant and McGrath (1990), predictors of the greatest need include the following characteristics:

More caregivers of mentally retarded women than men required respite care. Retarded sons were allowed freedom to venture into the community, reducing the need for respite; while caregivers of daughters with mental retardation tended to keep them at home to minimize the risk of abuse in the community, thus requiring need for respite.

146 | A GUIDE TO MENTAL RETARDATION

Older and/or retired caregivers, who often are widowed, rely less upon respite care because they have more time to devote to care and also appear to center their lives much more upon their son or daughter, who is frequently the only person remaining at home with them.

For a mentally retarded individual to successfully make the transition into adulthood, these important educational and vocational programs and their many components must be in place to provide support and resources.

As the programs continue to evolve and new ones develop, we come closer to recognizing the mentally retarded person's potential contribution to society. And there is no time that is any more important in the life of a mentally retarded individual than his or her aging-out years.

5

Adult Living

After the retarded person has made his or her way through the transitional process necessary to prepare him or her for the adult world, some issues will have been worked through and left behind, and some will remain. There will be other issues to face: some issues shared by the general population, and some that are specific to the individual.

The Developmentally Disabled as a Minority

Not until the Civil Rights Act of 1964, which benefited all minority groups, were persons with developmental disabilities considered full citizens and thereby entitled to all rights as citizens.

According to one agency, specific rights of handicapped persons include, but are not limited to, the following:

(1) Board and Care. Persons have the right to a normalized lifestyle; the right to choose their living situation; the right to a balanced and nutritious diet; the right to receive, own, and use personal belongings; the right to individualization within a community residence setting; the right to consider a residence as his or her home; the right to appropriate clothing for age and season, and the right to be involved in its selection; and the right to have enough grooming and personal hygiene supplies for his or her own use.

148 | A GUIDE TO MENTAL RETARDATION

(2) Communication. Persons have the right to communicate, associate, and meet privately with other individuals of their choice where this does not infringe on the rights of others; the right to receive visits from family, friends, and guardians and to make such visits; and the right to phone calls and letters to or from others.

(3) Health Services and Medical Care. Persons have the right to appropriate medical and dental care and the right, either personally or through a guardian, to a choice of physician or dentist; the right to general good health and to receive any special health or medical services needed because of his or her handicap or condition; and the right to a second medical opinion, such that no unnecessary or excessive medication will be given.

(4) Financial. Persons have the right to be gainfully employed; and the right to information regarding their financial status and assistance in the use of their resources.

(5) Activities. Persons have the right to participate in activities which are meaningful, appropriate, and productive; the right to participate in community/neighborhood activities, and to participate in planning these activities; and the right to engage in appropriate activities although some risk is involved.

(6) Services. Persons have the right to active programming; the right to their programming; the right to continuity of treatment; and to staff who are trained adequately to provide supervision, assistance, and guidance to all clients in a skillful, safe, and humane way with respect for personal dignity.

(7) Sexuality. Persons have the right to be informed about sexuality and available family planning services in the community: the right to express his or her sexuality within their ability to consent, as long as this does not infringe on others' rights; information about and regulation of conception; the right to carry a pregnancy to term or to have an abortion; and the right to marry and have a family.

(8) Education. Persons have the right to education to the fullest extent to which they are intellectually capable, provided through the regular channels of public education.

(9) Religion. Persons have the right to practice the religion or faith of their choice, through the method they choose, including the right not to participate.

(10) Voting. Persons have the right to register and vote, and to participate in activities that educate them in their civic responsibilities.

(11) Protection. Persons have the right to protection from neglect, abuse, maltreatment, and restraints; the right to guardianship or other legal forms of protective advocacy; the right to be protected from commercial or other exploitation and cruel or dehumanizing treatment; the right to confidentiality of their records; and the right to due process of law.

Legal Protection

Legal problems of institutionalized persons with mental retardation comprise a neglected area that is beginning to draw increased attention as institutional reform progresses (Patton et al. 1986). Three relatively new innovations — advocates, Human Rights Committees, and ombudsman services — are used to protect the rights of people who are developmentally disabled.

Advocacy Agencies

Examples of advocacy agencies for people with mental retardation as a class include the President's Committee on Mental Retardation, the Council for Exceptional Children, and the Association for Retarded Citizens (Patton et al. 1986). Agencies advocating on the individual level include state agencies, citizen advocates, and legally trained advocates (Patton et al. 1986).

Human Rights Committees (HRCs)

Human Rights Committees work within institutions and are designed to protect the rights of institutionalized persons with mental retardation. These committees review behavior management programs; investigate grievances, complaints, and allegations of rights violations; review research programs; investigate allegations of

150 | A GUIDE TO MENTAL RETARDATION

abuse and neglect; advocate and protect the rights of residents; and review resident care (Patton et al. 1986).

Ombudsman

This is a relatively new concept. An ombudsman is "one whose role is to protect the rights of individuals seeking services from government agencies and educational systems." While an advocate would be an outsider to an institution, an ombudsman works within the institution (Patton et al. 1986).

The following interview with a legal professional and advocate for developmentally disabled individuals, offers a more in-depth picture of advocacy.

Q: Describe your advocacy connection with the mentally retarded population.

I'm working with . . . Legal Services on a grant from the . . . State Commission on Quality of Care in a program called Protection and Advocacy for the Developmentally Disabled; it also serves other people with similar disabilities.

The federal government wrote a protection and advocacy bill that says that states who want to receive special federal funding have to set up a program that provides protection and advocacy. New York State decided to set up the commission and hired attorneys and placed them throughout the state.

Basically, what we do is sue the state to keep them in conformance with their own regulations. In other words, the state pays us to keep it in compliance with its own regulations — it's a monitoring device. It's an affirmative action program meant to keep the current state systems in compliance.

Q. Who becomes an advocate?

Our program requires a person to be an attorney — they have to be licensed and a member of the bar to practice. Otherwise, anybody who has any information or skills in the area can offer himself or herself as an advocate.

Adult Living | 151

Q: Parents are often the best advocates. Do you provide assistance to parents?

I've had parents who have come to my trainings — a four-day program that anyone can attend. It was started for parents who wanted to make themselves available to agencies in our region to go with parents to committee meetings and treatment planning meetings.

Many of these people are with agencies already, such as caseworkers for Developmental Disabilities Service Office (DDSO), Department of Social Services (DSS), private agencies, or independent living centers. There are advocates all over the place.

There are advocates out there who have their name in the phone book. Generally, the advocates who are freelancing are in the field of special education because there is more of a demand for them there, and more money available. Usually, the disabled child has a parent with an income. An adult with a disability may not have someone else's income to depend on.

Advocates for the adult population are not going to be freelancers; they're going to be the agency staff hired to represent them. There could be a caseworker for a person at ARC, for instance, and part of her job is to advocate for that person.

Q: What are some major issues faced in adulthood for persons with mental retardation or any other developmental disability that may require advocacy?

Generally, the mentally retarded person requires advocacy wherever he or she has any interaction or contact with the state. It could be the state licensing facility; it could be the transportation service; it could be a private consulting firm that provides services to the residential setting.

Whenever the person has contact with that agency and there's a conflict over what the agency is doing — like changing the person's placement, changing their job assignment, changing their transportation route — at any of those times they really need an advocate present to make sure that the individual's rights are being represented. An individual does have the right to make an objection to those kinds of placement changes and to those changes in their treatment plan.

152 | A GUIDE TO MENTAL RETARDATION

An advocate would be essential any time a disabled person can't articulate, or doesn't have the capacity to understand the laws protecting [disabled people]. For example, in one situation, they may be asked to move to a different residence, but don't want to make the move. The advocate can mediate on their behalf and ensure that the client's wishes are heard and respected. If the client doesn't have an advocate, the system is not really being used to the client's advantage.

Q: What is the role of the advocate in instances where the rights of the individual may go unmet or even unnoticed?

The advocate serves to educate, advocate, and work toward conflict resolution. For example, what happens when the client objects to a job change or a placement change? What happens when the client objects to a medication change? Sometimes there are things that the state may do to the client which could infringe upon that person's constitutional or civil rights.

However, there are separate legal questions about constitutional rights not to have one's privacy — one's person, one's chemical make-up — altered despite one's objection or without one's consent. The person's disability may prevent their understanding that they have constitutional or civil rights; they may not understand that those legal rights exist regardless of whether they are in the care and treatment of an agency. The agency in this case, because it's licensed by the state, cannot do anything to violate the individual's civil or constitutional rights — even though the agency believes that it is doing what it best.

If an agency, thinking that it is doing something clinically sound, approaches a client who is not capable of fully understanding his situation, the client may say "I have no problem." However, it is a legal violation to solicit consent from an individual who has not been judged competent by a court to give consent on his own behalf. Where there's any question of infringement on a person's civil or constitutional rights — such as medication changes or use of physical restraints — the facility is required to go to court with that individual to show whether that individual is or is not competent to give or deny consent.

Q: How is an advocate who is an attorney different from other advocates?

The advocate, in general, assists the person in making their way appropriately through the system. The attorney, on the other hand, is present solely for filing papers and dealing directly with the court.

You must have an attorney for anything that takes place in court. But the advocate who is not an attorney can be involved right from the beginning — can go to the treatment team meetings with the client and/or the parent; can discuss the question of medication and increased dosage with the client; made suggestions, for example, "Listen, are you sure this is what you want? These are the things that may end up happening to you. These are your options." Advocates can discuss legal options with the individual, from the individual's point of view. That advocate would then articulate the individual's position to the agency.

Q: Will an individual with mental retardation be an advocate for himself or herself?

Yes. This is called self-advocacy. There is a whole new trend — in [this state], at least — which basically is educational in nature. It tells clients: You have a right to this, and here is how you do it: You fill out this form. You go to this person and say, "I want this form filled out. I want to be able to smoke in my bedroom at night."

Q: With an advocate, is there the concern that the process will slow down?

That's a possibility. The clinicians probably would use that as an excuse. However, it has to be viewed from the point of view of the Constitution, which gives us rights and protections from people intruding on our privacy. If you respect those rights and protections enough, to wait until due process has been completed is a drop in the bucket.

154 | A GUIDE TO MENTAL RETARDATION

Q: What if it is difficult to determine whether the person agrees or disagrees with a recommendation?

If you're in a . . . licensed facility, there are very specific procedures for that. If you work in an agency and you meet up with a client on an issue that raises a constitutional or civil rights question, and you think the person does not have the capacity to give or deny consent, then you have to refer the individual to the Surrogate Decision-Making Committee in the facility. That committee is required to hire an outside expert to review the case, and to do an evaluation on the client to determine whether or not the individual has the capacity to give or deny consent.

Q: What happens if the individual is deemed unable to give consent?

Say, for example, the agency wants to have a female client's tubes tied, and they say that they have a clinical reason for doing this. If there is no guardian around, and the person is clearly too mentally retarded to understand the nature of the procedure, the State has to refer to the Surrogate Decision-Making Committee who then has to follow several procedures. If they ultimately decide that the individual, who may be communicating or responding as if to say, "No, I don't want surgery," is too mentally retarded to know the difference between what is good or bad for them, they then have to take that individual before a judge to establish if this person is capable of understanding the benefits and drawbacks of the surgery. The judge must establish whether, if they had the capacity, the individual would consent to the operation.

Human Rights: Between Talk and Action

Two experienced workers in a large agency for clients who are retarded talked about their experience and concerns with the important issue of human rights.

"Some rights issues are so obvious that they are readily enforced. For example, if an employee hits a client, they are in trouble immediately and are fired; they can even have legal charges brought against them. Other rights are not protected as readily, and this is not due to a lack of concern by workers but to the limited services provided.

"The right to privacy is a good example here. If a person lives in a group home with twelve other people they will have to have a roommate and share a bathroom with six others. This limits their privacy. It's not the same as for other citizens."

The limited capacity of adult programs for providing educational services is another factor that limits people's "right to an education." In a classroom with fifteen people and two staff, you're not going to be able to provide a person "with what they really need to progress in life."

Recent legislation emphasizes the rights of people who have developmental disabilities but some workers have expressed wariness: "I think the legislators are trying to say that people who are handicapped have as many rights as people who are not handicapped. And they've realized they've said this, and now we've agreed to it. But how it actually comes out in the wash is very different."

One experienced program director emphasizes: "When we look at providing our clients with the same rights as any adult, we are torn because they deserve adult rights but have the mental capacities of children. We can't say, 'They're adults, they have the responsibilities of adults, so let them decide and make mistakes for themselves.' Even with your own children, there are times when you just let your child learn from their mistakes. But there are times when you have to intervene: you don't want your child to go up and touch a wood stove. There's a delicate balance."

For the guardian to find a balance between protecting the client and allowing him to make mistakes is very difficult: "To respect people as adults, for them to have their own personhood and all of those rights, but at the same time protect them so that in making choices they don't hurt themselves — that's a very hard line to draw. And I think we're always trying to draw that line.

"Some people talk about total independence. I think for some people with mental retardation, it is definitely possible for them to live with very little support. But for many, many others, I don't know if we're ever going to reach that place. They may always need our help. We have to ask ourselves, 'How much can this person realistically decide on his or her own? And when does he or she need our help?' Again, it's a dilemma for us."

156 | A GUIDE TO MENTAL RETARDATION

What limits the choices, independence, integration, and productivity of persons with mental retardation? While the Medicaid Waiver offers to open doors for persons who are mentally retarded, the "old thinking" may leave workers feeling uncomfortable providing their consumers with new opportunities for choice and independence.

A recent conference introduced this new way of thinking, and asked participants to discuss their fears about the changes taking place in New York State (see Appendix A) and the obstacles in the present system which may impede the areas of choice, independence, integration, and productivity for consumers. The group, composed of workers from every level of care from administrators to social workers, psychologists, direct care workers, and residential staff, shared many useful and meaningful insights. Their discussion yielded lists of some of the things that interfere with serving consumers effectively:

Choices

— The individual's choice may conflict with areas of need designated by the treatment team

— The individual, either due to his or her development level or years of inopportunity, may have no understanding or practice of choice

— Having large groups/classes limits opportunities for one-to-one attention

— Not enough program staff

— Wasted time teaching unnecessary skills and/or unrealistic goals (for example, teaching money skills, but not supplying real opportunities to practice skills besides using a soda machine)

— New freedom will upset old routines

— Lack of resources and money

— Lack of individualized advocacy

— Lack of staff awareness — prejudice that consumers cannot make choices, cannot be independent (note: "staff" refers to workers at all levels)

— Lack of staff training in new ways of thinking and creativity in providing services to consumers

Adult Living | 157

— Pressures from guardians

— Lack of communication between agency programs, such as day treatment and residential programs (that is, skills need to be carried out in an integrated fashion from one setting to another)

— Consumers telling staff what staff want to hear

— Lack of job opportunities and program options from which to choose

Independence

— Rigid staff attitudes (for example, a client who wishes to walk to the door quickly may be told to sit down)

— Rigid programming

— Utilizing a classroom setting which may not be appropriate for adults

— Lack of trust based upon past behaviors (for example, fears of bringing consumer with a history of unpredictable, disruptive behavior out to the mall)

— Staff attitude: "It's just a job"

— Lack of staff and consumer motivation

— Homogeneous groups (people of equal levels of functioning) have no peer role models and, thus, may be disadvantageous

— Agency liability

— Dated belief systems: thinking that "old ways" are quicker and more efficient

Integration

— Large group size creates stigma

— Low direct-care staff ratio per group

— Limited transportation resources

— Infrequency of returning to settings where clients can develop relationships

— Receptivity of community

— Lack of bringing nonhandicapped people *into* the agency

— Staff perceptions: lack of ability to think of integration options

— Ideas not communicated or utilized in the past

158 | A GUIDE TO MENTAL RETARDATION

Productivity

— No reward for being productive
— Lack of understanding as to what productivity is (not only work production, but quality of life)
— Staff's preconceived ideas of leisure time and social events
— Self-awareness: lack of feedback on consumers' progress, whether in work production or with newly learned skills
— Not enough access to "real" activities
— Not enough staff reinforcement for positive, productive behaviors
— Failure to observe what really motivates consumers
— Lack of attention to possible *person* goals and future plans of consumers
— Lack of patience with consumers

From brain-storming sessions such as the one I attended, where workers at all levels are invited to come together to communicate fears and solutions, there is hope that the consumer will benefit in the end.

Impact of Deinstitutionalization

Deinstitutionalization has been described as a movement "dedicated to the dignity of individuals" with the basic aim being to improve the quality of life for people who are retarded (Bachrach 1981 in Emerson 1985). Alternative community-based services were implicitly mandated to provide the support necessary to help people with retardation enter society's mainstream.

Is deinstitutionalization really good for everyone? A program director remarks: "The community still doesn't accept the idea that people who are mentally retarded belong in the community. But is deinstitutionalization really the right thing for the clients? For many it was. But there were many others who really like the institutions; they've lost a family."

One such person was uncovered during their screening process: "One person had lived in a large institution for fifty years. She had the same roommate for the past forty years; there were people that she considered her family and she felt happy there. Would it be right, then, to yank this person from people she loved only to put her into a community that she didn't know, a house she didn't know, and people she didn't know, and have to say goodbye to her 'family'?"

One experienced physician comments: "I had a colleague who worked at the Willowbrook State School from the 1940s through the 1970s. While supportive of the reforms, this doctor was saddened at the loss of interpersonal relations ensuing from the complex post-Willowbrook legislation. There were many staff who genuinely loved the patients and made them part of their lives. They were unable to continue doing so with the new rules that monitored every aspect of contact with the Willowbrook clients. He felt that a great deal of abuse had been prevented, but something very intangible, and very beautiful, had been lost."

Social Issues in Adulthood

Public Acceptance

Probably one of the hardest issues to deal with for the person with retardation is acceptance by peers, coworkers, bosses, and the many other persons with whom he will come into contact. While the disability creates its own inherent limitations, to be labeled or stigmatized creates difficulties that can wound much deeper.

"Public acceptance and understanding," one author notes, "are interrelated processes which are crucial for the successful and active integration of retarded adults into our communities" (Patton et al. 1986). Still, once in the community, many persons with mental retardation encounter resistance and discrimination in employment, housing, education, and public service.

One staff person gives this illustration: "If you ever want to see it in action, go to a public hearing when a group home is going to be built in a town and listen to the panic and the perceptions expressed. You think, 'Is this the 1990s or the 1890s?' We were building a house in one community and had to go to a public hearing. Who else is required to go to a public hearing when they want to buy a house? But if I have a developmental disability, my advocate has to go and defend my rights in front of the town

160 | A GUIDE TO MENTAL RETARDATION

board. This in itself is a reflection of the archaic and isolationist attitudes of the public."

Overcoming Public Attitudes

Fortunately, the initial fears and reactions which have existed for so long, and which have gone through many different changes, can be prevented or changed. Most fears stem from a lack of public understanding of mental retardation. As one author writes: "Negative attitudes and fears concerning [individuals with developmental disabilities] frequently result from ignorance. Low expectations of the retarded and the fears associated with them often dissolve when 'normal' individuals meet retarded persons and see their abilities and potential" (Patton et al. 1987).

"When I go out to the store," one worker explains, "the clerks in the store get very flustered because they're not used to talking with someone they can't understand right away; they're not used to seeing someone who looks different.

"I think it's changing as more and more people live down the street from someone who has a developmental disability. They are used to seeing them and this is generating a positive change."

A number of subtle and not-so-subtle attitudes exist toward persons with retardation even today. A few of these are listed below, followed by a few illuminating facts (Schalock 1983).

Misconception #1: "Developmentally disabled persons are childlike." The truth is that many persons with disabilities cannot be distinguished from 'normal' people. Furthermore, disabled individuals often succeed in social and interpersonal interactions, and their mental and social age measurements do not take into account the person's learning experience or functioning level.

Often, people with mental retardation can be noticeably suggestible. This is partially due to expectations of failure, which causes the person to depend on other's judgment (Sternlicht 1977 in Schalock 1983). Also, their affectionate behavior, mistrust, and/or fear, as one researcher explains, may result from social deprivation (Schulman 1980 in Schalock 1983).

One man tells this story: "At one time I held the same misconception because of my lack of exposure to persons with milder

Adult Living | 161

forms of retardation. One day, however, as I changed my schedule around to accommodate two gentlemen who enjoy smoking their pipes, we ended up sitting in the cafeteria where people from an adjoining workshop were having their lunch. My pipe-smoking friends and I talked freely with one woman who, at first, I thought to be a staff member from the workshop; she was as articulate, funny, and pleasant as she could be. Later I found out that she was not staff. At that moment, I learned something."

Another staff member noted that treating people with mental retardation like children often meets the needs of the caregiver more than the needs of the recipient. "A common issue question is "Why is it wrong to hug so-and-so?' It's important to try to get the idea across that this person doesn't have to always be limited by the situation they're in right now. Maybe months or years from now they will be living out in the world. You wouldn't want this person walking up to some stranger and hugging him. If you had a brother or sister who is forty-five, you wouldn't want them going around hugging people. Why not teach appropriate things; the same things you and I would do?

"There's a parent who talks to me about her 'baby girl.' Well, her 'baby girl' is forty-five, and she refers to the other program clients as 'kids in the classroom.' Her identity is that of mother, but her child doesn't act childlike. This parent's whole identity is invested in being the mom and caregiver of a 'baby girl.'

"While these people are developmentally delayed, we are not always aware of how much we contribute to keeping them emotionally delayed by the way we treat them."

Misconception #2: "Group homes lower adjacent property values." Some neighbors silently harbor or openly express this fear. The truth is that property values in areas with group homes neither increase nor decrease (Wolpert 1978 in Schalock 1983). Furthermore, the proximity to group homes does not affect a property's market value, nor does the existence of a group home generate a higher degree of neighborhood property turnover (Novak and Heal 1980 in Schalock 1983).

One town board member brought up a fascinating point, contrary to the above belief: He said that "if a family moved into town with three kids, that would cost the town so much in tax-

162 | A GUIDE TO MENTAL RETARDATION

funded services: education, transportation, school buses, etc. A family with three kids costs the town a lot more in taxes than a group home."

Misconception #3: "Persons with developmental disabilities are better off in institutions than they are in the community." Community programs have been proved to increase self-esteem, socialization, and independence for persons with disabilities. In contrast, institutions often involve regimentation, limited choices, and a lack of privacy (Robinson and Robinson 1976 in Schalock 1983). In addition, they tend to reinforce dependency, compliance, and introversion (Thompson 1977 in Schalock 1983).

"You'd have to go into an institution and see how the system works," one individual explains. "I can remember a time when I tried to help a woman attend church services. She lives on the institution grounds, the church was on the institution grounds, and she was in a wheelchair. But because of the red tape around providing transportation for this woman, for months she couldn't go to a church less than a mile away. Sure, she could have been pushed in her wheelchair in warm weather. But an army of administrators and people from outside agencies were fighting this battle to get that woman a mere thousand yards and back on a Sunday morning. This is the stuff of someone's life in an institution."

"A more beneficial situation," another worker adds, "would be to feed all of the money directly to the clients, without having this huge administrative structure to accommodate.

"The best system is to offer family care or small houses with this money. You would do all of your day treatment right at the house just as you would in a normal situation. Even if you just rotate your staff it wouldn't matter. The individuals would get out of the house everyday; they would get their six hours of active programming — not necessarily inside the house.

"You now have one house with one electric bill and so on. You wouldn't need porter maintenance, there wouldn't be tremendous utility bills, there wouldn't be sky-high insurance rates. This would be the most normalizing, the most cost-effective situation."

While cost efficiency is one point, researchers also find that persons who are raised at home are generally superior intellectually and socially to institutionally reared persons (Kimble, Garmezy, and Zigler 1980 in Schalock 1983).

Misconception #4: "Persons with development disabilities present a threat to the community." The fact is that persons with mental retardation do not have a higher incidence of delinquency or crime, and the frequency of sexual delinquency is not more evident (Friedman 1977, Hart 1978 in Schalock 1983).

"Usually there is an implication that people with mental retardation will be unpredictable and possibly violent: a threat to their children, their pets, the public. People often have these strange misconceptions.

"A big issue for one group home in the planning stage was that the neighbor had little kids. This was *made* to be an issue: it's assumed because I have Down syndrome and I'm short and have a round face, that I'm going to molest kids. Yet I could have just been released from prison for child molestation and I don't even have to go to a public hearing. I could buy the house next door, and who would know?

"People were also outraged because the house had a swimming pool. They would say, 'How can you let these people move into a place with a swimming pool?' I would respond, 'How do you know that everybody who is going to live here isn't a champion swimmer?' But if I had a two-year-old, it's very unlikely that my two-year-old could swim. In this case, the town board isn't going to make a fuss about me moving in."

We do, however, see situations where individuals with mental retardation may pose a threat to themselves. "The behaviors that we may see aren't a mystery when we view the history that most of these people have had," one worker elaborates.

"I have seen very normal kids — children who have been born perfectly normal — who are understimulated in orphanages, just as people have been understimulated in institutions. I have seen these children rocking, banging their heads against their cribs — anything to keep stimulus coming in from the outside. If they do not get enough stimulation, they give it to themselves.

"This kind of self-stimulation keeps the individual alive — because infants can die without a certain level of stimulation. In essence, this is a healthy attempt at surviving. What happens later is

164 | A GUIDE TO MENTAL RETARDATION

that this self-stimulation can become inappropriate — self-abuse. Now, instead of banging against the crib, rocking, sucking their thumb, or doing whatever kids need to do to stay alive, we see them hitting themselves. And when we see them doing things like that, it is very difficult for us to understand. It is especially difficult for the inexperienced to understand these kinds of behaviors.

"One thing we need to realize is that these behaviors are an extension of the environment in which these people were raised. It is not something inherent in those who are mentally retarded or autistic or disabled in any way. It is a function of their need to stay alive."

Misconception #5: "Mental retardation is usually a hereditary condition and is not likely to occur in the typical family." The truth is that there are over 200 causes of mental retardation (see chapter 1). Retardation may be the result of any of the following: postnatal infection and/or trauma; damage to the developing central nervous system; infection and intoxication which can damage the fetus; exposure to rubella in the womb, which can affect 10% to 85% of babies (Schalock 1983).

Misconception #6: "Persons with developmental disabilities are incapable of becoming productive members of society." More and more exposure to the achievements of persons with mental retardation are provided on television and in the news. One commercial developed by McDonald's shows a retarded employee, Michael, proudly telling how he appreciates having the opportunity to provide a service to his community.

Employment rates, broken down by developmental levels, provide another illuminating picture: For persons with mild retardation, 87% of males and 33% of females are employed; for persons with moderate retardation, 12% of males and 12% of females are employed. However, although the success stories demonstrate the capabilities of the majority of persons with disabilities, as of 1979, 690,000 adults with mental retardation were without work, while about 400,000 could be gainfully employed if appropriate services were available (Schalock 1983).

Misconception #7: "Persons with developmental disabilities are incapable of learning." In truth, persons with developmental disabilities demonstrate a wide range of learning ability. Even persons with profound handicaps can develop self-help and simple communication skills. For example, there is one woman with profound retardation who demonstrates a remarkable number of communication signs in an employment setting.

As one worker points out, "There will be times when people I may expect the least from will come out with things that they picked up in spite of us."

Such examples abound: "One woman had a boyfriend who was in the hospital, and he was dying. We were concerned: should we take her to see her boyfriend? What will she do in the hospital? There were a lot of questions. We finally concluded that we couldn't make the decision for her. We talked with her, and she went to the hospital, and she was great! She was good for him; the nurses were impressed. And nobody knew that she had it in her."

"There was a woman who was taken to the hospital when a classmate was sick. This woman tends to be very loud and inappropriate. But she was wonderful in the hospital. She was perfectly appropriate. She would say, 'I feel sorry for you. How do you feel? You'll feel better. Don't worry.' She was completely appropriate."

"We don't realize how much of our own preoccupations and prejudices we bring into a situation, even though we're trained in the field. Training is not always an advantage. We tend, especially when we work with large groups, to characterize the groups as having this range of abilities; and when we see people constantly exceed that range, we are surprised."

"It has to do with the expectations," a program supervisor explains. "In this field, our expectations are generally very, very low. We say that the person is mentally retarded and we put that person in a group of mentally retarded people. Our system makes no demands on them, and therefore there are no positive expectations.

"For example, one new staff member sat in on lunch with a group of seniors. She wasn't used to the situation, and she saw the people just sitting in their seats with their lunch boxes in front of them; nobody moved. 'Come on, guys,' she said, 'go ahead and eat.' She then realized that the classroom staff were opening all of the lunch boxes and getting the sandwiches out, and so she suggested letting the clients do it themselves. While the program

166 | A GUIDE TO MENTAL RETARDATION

therapist actually responded very well, it was as if the concept of letting these people do what they can for themselves was totally unique. It was an expectation that these people could not even open their own lunch boxes."

Another professional who came into the field fairly inexperienced remembers feeling that "people who had worked in this field longer had developed a line of thinking which had become rigid. As a new person in the field, I would think, 'Why not do this?' After a while, I would hit barriers; my motivation would die, and the new ideas were no longer there. Now I see new people entering the field with the same hopeful attitude that I had. And I think, 'I had those ideas once.' "

"If everyone is more involved, the people are getting something out of it, they're more alert, they're happier, and they have increased self-esteem. In one classroom, everyone has something to do almost all day long. Those people are active and busy. This teacher is a unique person who knows how to get twelve people to build on each other's strengths and get each person to participate.

"Our agency, at present, provides no training or structure for these people beyond the limits of when someone grabs your hair, what to do if there's a fire in the wastebasket, how to protect yourself from hepatitis — those kinds of issues which are negative-based. They're already setting up a whole list of expectations right there: that these people are difficult; that they're going to harm you; that if you try to save them you may lose your job. There are lots of negative messages sent in the training we provide at the on-set of a new worker's experience.

"Unless you inspire the staff and train them to keep dispelling their own expectations and provide the kind of structure and resources for them to take off, it's not going to happen. A special education teacher goes through six years of college and an internship and they have very strict lesson plans. What do you require in a day treatment program? Not that much."

Misconception #8: "Persons with mental retardation are clumsy, abnormal, dull, and helpless." When college students were asked to distinguish persons with mental retardation from persons with mental illness, the students clearly distinguished the two (Caruso and Hodapp 1988). However, according to the poll, persons with mental retardation are still perceived as clumsy (having motor problems), abnormal (having physical defects and medical problems), dull (being slow learners with low I.Q.s), and helpless (unable to cope or function in society).

"Some people view *all* people with developmental retardation as having severe or profound retardation," noted one worker. "They don't realize the cognitive differences that exist within this population, and don't recognize that some people are able to maintain competitive employment at the local college or hospital, whereas others need the intensive support offered in a day treatment program."

Levels of Stress

Adult living requires the ability to deal with daily stresses that will arise. Such stress can create the energy one needs to get through tough times and tough decisions, but may at times become so overwhelming that we need to stand back for a short while. However we may handle these situations, we at least have some understanding about these feelings and may even have a successful way to cope, given what we have learned in our own lives.

The interpretations and experiences of stress for the person with retardation are different. In fact, people with mental retardation experience more, rather than less, stress than their nonhandicapped peers (Deutsch 1989). Some believe that this "heightened level of fearfulness and anxiety" may result from having been sheltered from everyday stress and opportunities (Levine 1985).

Sources of Stress

From the perspective of the individual with retardation, stress may emerge from three sources (Deutsch 1989). First, situations that are typically stressful to the general population will, naturally, be stressful to someone who has mental retardation. Events such as changing jobs, moving, death of a family member or friend can create overwhelming anxieties in any person.

However, from the perspective of the individual with mental retardation, who has poorer coping skills and is generally not as well prepared for similar life events, the level of anxiety and stress will increase considerably. As one author notes: "It is interesting

168 | A GUIDE TO MENTAL RETARDATION

that these people who experience particular difficulty in dealing with stress generally receive less preparation and less coping-skills training than the rest of society. It is not uncommon, for example, for someone with mental retardation to have very little notice when changing homes or jobs. These people have very little input into the direction of their lives, yet are expected to 'handle' these dramatic life changes often without support" (Deutsch 1989).

Research in the area illustrates the importance of providing persons with mental retardation *while growing up* with a variety of experiences to aid in their ability to handle stress (Levine 1985). For example, adults with retardation who are employed — whether competitively or in a sheltered workshop setting — are less likely to respond with anxiety than unemployed individuals with mental retardation. In addition, adults with disabilities who are socially active and gregarious are less likely to be anxious to situations than are individuals who have been socially isolated.

A second source of stress for the individual with mental retardation is the ordinary situation which is typically handled with ease by the general population. Since these individuals generally have poor coping skills, they frequently misread social situations, and the anxiety they feel can have a negative impact on their self-esteem. As an example, going out to dinner and then to the movies for someone who typically has limited opportunities to participate in these activities can create stress; the person with retardation may feel uncomfortable that he is different from other people encountered in public situations.

Individuals with mental retardation must also deal with stresses which are unique to them, often involving a combination of internal and external events. For example, one gentleman who is retarded tells how he often compares himself with nonhandicapped people, resulting in his rating himself negatively. As he compared himself with the expectations of many adults, he wondered if he'd ever be able to accomplish things such as dating and marriage, handling his own money, making his own decisions, owning and driving a car, living independently — events which symbolize independence, adulthood, and normality. The truth is that many adult expectations fostered in our society are not achieved by most adults with mental retardation.

Training Programs

While some persons with mental retardation, through opportunities in work and social interactions, are able to obtain skills at handling stressful situations, others — particularly those individuals functioning at lower levels — may require specialized training which, as research has demonstrated, can be acquired through systematic training (as expressed in Griffiths 1990a).

Historically, while significant progress has been made in vocational, domestic, and educational skills training to enhance the lives of persons with developmental disabilities, significantly less emphasis has been given to the teaching of skills that assure successful emotional and social integration for persons with handicaps until only recently (Griffiths 1990a).

Social skills can be acquired through systematic training; however, such training is often ineffective because the skills are taught in small "chunks" devoid of the appropriate social context (Griffiths 1990b). To assure a more successful outcome, it is suggested that all social skills training should: incorporate the teaching of valued behaviors; occur in a social context; occur in a natural social setting; involve teaching individuals to evaluate social situations; and use training techniques that promote generalizations to the natural environment and build social independence (Griffiths 1990b).

Demonstrating Competence

Demonstrating competence and maintaining self-esteem may be crucial issues in the lives of adults with mental retardation (Edgerton 1971 in Levine 1985). Those individuals who have worked and/or been active socially have increased opportunities for learning how to cope with self-esteem problems.

Persons with mental retardation can learn to manage anxiety, largely as an outcome of meaningfully experiencing and coping with normal, everyday living and problem-solving (Levine 1985). All too often, however, they are not provided with the opportunities and the experiences from which to develop a sense of competence.

170 | A GUIDE TO MENTAL RETARDATION

"At this time, I don't think we're that skilled in terms of providing clients with opportunities to get those basic skills. It's not that different from what we experience ourselves: To know how to do something gives us a tremendous amount of self-esteem."

Staff need to remember to work at a slower pace. We can't look at our own satisfaction as being reflective of their satisfaction. Progress may seem slow, but to them they are advancing in leaps and bounds.

"What we as staff want to do is fulfill our need to write goals, filling out the paperwork. That is what currently drives us, rather than asking: 'What does this person need; what does this person like?'

"If an individual — a child or an adult with a developmental disability — wants to do something, and you show him the joy of doing it, then he'll take care of the rest; he may even learn faster than we could imagine."

Few would argue that the ability to move about in one's community is essential. It helps a person get to know other people and places, as well as aids in his or her developing a sense of personal control over one's surroundings.

This ability to travel is not easily attainable for persons with mental retardation, however. Most do not have a driver's license; instead, they must depend upon other people — parents, caretakers — for getting them around. There are those who, because they lack skills in reading, telling time, or determining correct change, are unable to use public transportation systems. Physical disabilities, such as those resulting from cerebral palsy, are the most limiting of all.

As one researcher notes: "Deinstitutionalization does not automatically provide all of the answers; some professionals and administrators have not realized that the transition from institutional/dependent behavior to more independent behavior is not achieved simply by moving people into the community" (Robinson, Griffith, McComish, and Swasbrook 1984).

Fortunately, many educational, vocational, and residential programs for persons with mental retardation now include instruction in street safety and mobility skills. For persons with milder forms of mental retardation, skills needed to use public transportation, ask strangers for help, find the police, and use money are all included in travel training, along with social skills and the etiquette of being a passenger, recognizing buildings, and using the telephone (Patton et al. 1986).

Robinson et al. (1984) demonstrates the effectiveness of travel training in the use of buses, finding that subjects learned the necessary skills, while maintaining their performance for at least one year.

While advances have been made in many areas of enabling persons with mental retardation to enjoy mobility, more advances need to be made.

Only recently, with the Americans with Disabilities Act, has legislative action related to mobility taken place. The opportunity of increased mobility is described by one worker: "Persons who are developmentally disabled are, in essence, riding on the coat tails of new federal legislation. It was not designed specifically for people who are developmentally disabled. However, a lot of our clients are also physically disabled.

"What this act is saying is that within a couple of years all existing public buildings are going to have to have to be handicap accessible: ramps, for example. In addition, public transportation will have some accessible units in place, such as wheelchair lifts.

"Communication systems will have to be revamped. We probably are going to have telephone communication that will show pictures as well. If one is not able to hear over the phone, signing or lip reading can be used.

"There is a definite timetable set up for these changes to take place. Accessible transportation has to be furnished by the year 1996, and new public buildings are required by law to be accessible. Eventually, even if it takes a few more years, the changes will occur across the entire country.

"The Civil Rights Act of 1964, which most people don't associate with developmental disabilities, took a look at the way people were being discriminated against and helped establish programs to remedy those situations. The Americans with Disabilities Act also advances the cause of the disabled population's mobility and accessibility."

One worker recalls observing some of the changes which have already taken place: "I go camping a lot. I recently noticed an addition up at the campground — the whole new addition is totally handicap accessible — down to the beach itself, and even into the woods. Even picnicking is accessible."

172 | A GUIDE TO MENTAL RETARDATION

While the Americans with Disabilities Act seems promising, one has to question whether it is a realistic proposition financially, especially for those buildings requiring modification.

"There is the cost factor," one worker responds. "What's right to do versus what's possible to do — you can run into trouble. I've heard that with regular school systems they're being pushed to the very limit of their budgets. And then all of a sudden someone is saying that they have to put an elevator in the school. These are difficult issues.

"For a long time, this country thought that there was no limit to money. And now we're starting to see that maybe there is a limit, and what this might mean. Again, these are hard, hard issues, and people are going to be hurt by the answers."

"The federal government is able to enforce this by attaching incentives to community businesses and schools," one worker adds. "If they don't provide means of accessibility for handicapped individuals, schools don't get federal aid; the Department of Transportation doesn't receive money if they don't convert their buses. So people are motivated to provide these things."

Ideally, state and federal legislation regarding accessibility issues offers hope for improving the quality of life for individuals with disabilities of all kinds. Working out the funding problems and balancing the needs of all members of the community remain an ongoing challenge.

Quality of Life

How satisfied are you with your life? To consider this, we look at the various parts of our lives: family, friendships, education, the place we live in, and our jobs. I realize that, while there may be limitations, the quality of my life, for the most part, is a result of what I have been able to put into it; if I wish to change matters, there are always means that I can take to change my situation.

For persons with mental retardation, however, much of their quality of life is determined, not by them, but by the family, caretakers, policymakers, and staff around them, some of whom are very loving and sensitive to the individual. However, there exist many individuals whose desires and needs go unmet, or are misinterpreted by the caretaker.

Research evaluating the quality of life for the individual with mental retardation considers two variables. First are social indicators, such as community participation or exclusion, power, autonomy, social networks, life events, activity patterns, lifestyles, and role functioning. The second and most important variable, person satisfaction, is an area that, unfortunately, has been seriously neglected. As one researcher comments, "Failure to canvas client opinion is to continue to condone the exclusion of retarded people from taking active participant roles in decisions affecting their own lives" (Emerson 1985).

In deinstitutionalization, some of the placements for persons with retardation clearly would not be seen as adequate or satisfying to anyone. According to one researcher, "All too often, community services conspire to re-enact the very same institutional processes of ensuring the physical and social isolation and stigmatization of handicapped persons, maintaining the degrading asymmetrical power relationships between residents and staff, and encouraging dependency and regimentation" (Emerson 1985).

According to Emerson's findings, persons living in the community "still interact mainly with other handicapped persons or paid staff, experience loneliness as a considerable problem, continue to be excluded from the labor force, experience little autonomy, spend endless hours in useless inactivity, and have little experience of everyday aspects of community living." Bercovici (1981 in Emerson 1985) further adds that "many deinstitutionalized persons with mental retardation are not, and do not, perceive themselves to be living in the normal community. . . . these persons may be seen, instead, as inhabitants of a physically segregated and culturally distinct social system."

"As for all individuals," another author states, "the development of a positive sense of self, so critical for daily living, is a lifelong endeavor for mentally retarded individuals. The stakes are a bit higher for them, and the cards are slightly stacked against them" (Patton et al. 1986).

Friendships

Few people would deny the importance of having friends in one's life to add to the safety, intimacy, self-esteem, and general enjoyment of living. While people with mental retardation want and

174 | A GUIDE TO MENTAL RETARDATION

need friendships like everyone else, they are often denied opportunities to form relationships or to develop skills necessary to interact socially with others (Patton et al. 1986).

Many factors influence the degree to which persons with mental retardation are able to acquire and maintain friends (Patton et al. 1986). Their exposure to peers may be limited because they live and work in sheltered or isolated environments. They typically lack a history of socializing events such as school clubs or parties that help to develop and refine personal skills.

Sometimes, by the very nature of their hunger for attention, some individuals with mental retardation may come on as overly affectionate which can repel people — potential friends. As I walk through a day treatment or workshop environment, it is rare that I, or any other staff member, can reach the other side of a room without an overwhelming draw of attention and affection from the people in the room. The desire to give them the attention is there — sometimes the impulse is to provide them with too much.

Current research interests in friendship reflect the importance of community projects for adults with developmental disabilities (Clegg and Standen 1991). Based upon a survey by Halpern, Close, and Nelson (1986 in Clegg et al. 1991), personal relationships are rated as the second most difficult aspect of living independently by people with developmental disabilities.

The opportunities to form and maintain friendships for individuals who come from an institutional background are grim. One sensitive worker talks about the situation in which a person has lived through the coldness of an institution: "I always think of the tendency of these people to form relationships with staff as another form of a survival mechanism, and an extremely appropriate way to get oneself set up — in other words, to thrive and to survive in that environment.

"You realize, on some level, that you are all dependent and identify with the caregiver, and then you immediately start to relate to them and build a relationship with them. In this way, you become a person; you become known.

"It is also a way to protect yourself from the other people in the room. You don't know how to relate to those other people: They're probably going to be uprooted and replaced by someone else, and you've learned not to trust them overall as a population.

You've learned how to identify that these people are different from you, that these people over here probably won't hurt you, but these people over there . . . you're not too sure. This person sitting next to you who never says anything, all of a sudden may begin to scream or hit you. You learn, very quickly, not to trust those kind of people. You would in any situation."

One worker asks if being in a homogeneous group hinders the development of natural relationships. "Considering where I work, at times I wonder when teaching relationship skills and appropriate interactions with peers: is there an extra hurdle created in trying to make one person with mental retardation make friends with another person with mental retardation? As opposed to providing the disabled person with a smaller setting — like family care — where he or she can interact and learn more normalized skills through the modeling of higher functioning people? In our setting, it seems as if we're forcing them to make relationships with people who may not be able to reciprocate."

Can these people, who historically have been grouped together, learn to trust each other? "In an institutional setting or classroom setting, it's very difficult," one worker responds.

"One of the ways you can help is to have the teacher participate with people on an equal level in accomplishing something. For instance, if you're going to make a meal, you all get involved in making the meal, and you encourage people to rely on each other and learn to trust each other in the context of an activity. We are all going to do something, but we're all equal in the sense that we all have to participate for the task to reach completion.

"I've seen it done in our senior section where, for example, Cheryl and Sue will be responsible for doing a task together: going into the kitchen together, washing the cups, putting them in the rack, and then bringing them back to the classroom. At this point, now that they've done this, they are allowed to do this on their own. Now they're in the kitchen, and they're talking and chatting like two girlfriends. And they're learning to trust each other; they're learning to do things together; they're interacting."

"All too often we set up artificial interactions," another worker comments. "For example, asking someone to go over and shake so-and-so's hand. What does that mean to that person? We shake all sorts of people's hands who we could care less about!

176 | A GUIDE TO MENTAL RETARDATION

It's just a social custom; it has no meaning behind it. It seems as if we're just making them go through the motions, and then that's it; it seems to stop there.

"You have to give them meaningful ways to interact. Just as you would build any friendship, it has to start with trust and interaction, and it has to be reality-based. It can't be artificial."

Most agencies, at present, emphasize goalwork: The individual requires a goal to increase his social interaction. "That's the problem with these so-called goals that are written to increase, for example, sharing an activity with a peer," one worker explains. "The activity, however, is completely meaningless to both people, It's a busy activity which has no point to it.

"And neither person has any emotional investment in the activity, or gets any pleasure out of it — they get absolutely nothing out of it. And it doesn't increase their self-esteem. Furthermore, the activity may be changed every day, so they don't actually learn to build relationships or obtain any sense of accomplishment or connection with another individual."

But some programs have been successful at group building and social skills training through, for example, music therapy. One worker tells the following story: "Many months ago when I was still fairly new to this field, I was walking through the hall and heard our music therapist involved with a small group of individuals. On a laptop piano, he was playing a simple song to which everyone sang and accompanied with percussive instruments. As the months went by, I continued to hear this song — over and over — and thought how irritating it was becoming. I wondered about the purpose of playing a simple song over and over. Later, I learned not to question the rationale behind another's profession; the explanation was, itself, simple and enlightening."

"A lot of staff thought it was ridiculous how monotonous it was to deal with the same song all of the time," a fellow worker recalls. "He would get people in the room three times a week and they'd do the same song for three months, four months, five months, until every staff person in the building could sing that song spontaneously; you could hear it in your sleep.

"However, what happened was that if you went and sat in that group, these people, by this time, knew a routine, and they felt good about it. They knew that the drum was going to come to them, then they'd beat the drum and say their name, then when the music went BOOM, they knew to stop beating the drum, and hand the drum to the next person. They learned something.

"Not only did they learn something, but they kept repeating and reinforcing the fact that they knew how to do something. And they felt great about themselves. I can do this. I know exactly how to do this. I know what is coming up. I know what is expected of me. I know everything about this.' But we don't give them enough opportunities to do this.

"As a group, they would start to pull together, because they all knew the routine and they all began to trust each other and there was an interaction — they had to rely on each other to pass the drum.

"I think there's particularly a lot of success in music therapy because people really do enjoy music. However, it's not used enough in as many ways as it could. For example, using the song 'He's Got the Whole World in His Hands,' it was hard for people to see the song as a teaching tool. But you get to identify people in your class and sing a song that most people knew. Not only do they feel really good because they know that song and they feel good when they sing, but they get to know each other's names. You can then expand that activity to the limits of whatever the group wants to get involved with.

"One day, as an activity, I played a rhythm and people got up and danced. Soon, groups of people got up to dance. Pretty soon, everyone was up and dancing. My hands were sore after I had played for twenty to twenty-five minutes. But it was almost like this cumulative effect. This drumming — this rhythm — is now a part of them, and these people got up and started to move who wouldn't budge in the first five minutes. After a while, people are interacting, and then they're laughing and feeling loose."

Sexuality

Years of Misunderstanding

Historically, society, in its need to feel comfortable and safe, had considered the population of mentally retarded individuals as non

178 | A GUIDE TO MENTAL RETARDATION

sexual. Administrative policies for persons with mental retardation in the area of sexuality, as recently as the early 1960s, instead had focused on areas such as legal consent relevant to issues of sexual abuse. However, little focus had been given to ethical and psychological implications of sexual expression among these people (Abramson, Parker, and Weisberg 1988).

Hall (1974 in Abramson et al. 1988) believes that public morality served as the basis for sexual restrictions often placed upon mentally retarded individuals. In addition, despite the objective to eliminate sexual abuse, there still existed an abundance of historical legislation and institutional policy that was designed to nullify sexual expression among the mentally retarded individuals of that day.

For example, for many decades such individuals were portrayed as moral pariahs (Braginsky and Braginsky 1971 in Abramson et al. 1988). Furthermore, mentally retarded individuals were often presumed genetically defective and targeted for state-enforced sterilization (Abramson et al. 1988). The trend to judicially condone sterilization on the belief that "mental deficiency accelerates sexual impulses and tendencies toward crime to a harmful degree" was still evident in the late 1960s and early 1970s (Abramson et al. 1988).

"People with mental retardation are one of the most scrutinized groups in our society," expresses one worker. "Frankly, it is quite incredible that there is not more acting out, more illegal activity, and more assaultive behaviors. If you or I were scrutinized and controlled to the same extent as the people we work with, I think we would have a very difficult time controlling some of our impulses.

"Our society isolated these people — put them out in the sticks — away from population centers. They were seen as either 'touched by God' or 'touched by the devil.' Either notion is far off the mark."

Since these early years of naiveté and fear, this position has been reversed, shifting from protecting society to protecting the rights and interests of all individuals. Many prejudices and fears may still exist in the community. Even within state agencies, those who serve persons with developmental disabilities reveal difficulty accepting these individuals as sexual beings.

Adult Living | 179

Myths about Sexuality and Mental Retardation

"The studies show sexual development of persons with mental deficiencies is greatly affected and determined by the myths, concerns, and ignorance of parents, professionals, and the general public" (Patton et al. 1986). Some common myths, which may still exist today, include the following (Patton et al. 1986):

People with mental retardation

— are not interested in sex;

— are oversexed;

— lack the ability to comprehend information regarding their sexuality;

— lack the ability to responsibly control their sexual desires;

— have enough difficulties without becoming involved with the risks of a sexual relationship;

—will have mentally retarded children; and

— cannot adequately care for a child.

As a result of these fears, many persons with mental retardation have been "sheltered" from sex information, references to love or dating, and opportunities to interact with members of the opposite sex (Patton et al. 1986).

The accumulated effects of such myths on the individuals can often be personally devastating, and counseling may be needed. Counseling with the developmentally handicapped, however — while often difficult and frustrating due to problems in communication and differences in life experience between counselor and client — is compounded even more when dealing with sexual issues. The individual may, for example, be afraid of discussing or disclosing information for which he or she has received punishment in the past.

One researcher involved in sex counseling for the developmentally disabled at York Central Hospital identifies some problem areas that this population often exhibits. First, many individuals show a disturbance in their self-concept. "We find that clients reveal not so much a poor self-concept, but a confused concept" (Hingsburger 1987).

Second, individuals experience isolation from their peers. Most clients have a primary counselor assigned to them for overall case coordination. Since they are powerful individuals who live,

180 | A GUIDE TO MENTAL RETARDATION

work, care for, and celebrate with the client, "it is not surprising that these staff members often become more important to them than the clients' own natural peers. What exists is a 'social service blanket' wrapped around the developmentally handicapped client, protecting him from outside relationships" (Hingsburger 1987).

Third, individuals will internalize inaccurate sexual knowledge. Some may be simply rote information, where the meaning behind the words or responses they elicit are not truly understood. In addition, the myths that exist about sexuality and the developmentally disabled may have been passed on to them, possibly creating a devastating effect on their self-image. As Hingsburger (1987) explains: "One of the most prevalent myths is that 'developmentally handicapped people are more likely to have developmentally handicapped children.' When this explanation is presented to the clients as a reason for remaining nonsexual, it may actually convey the message, 'If you have sex, you will get pregnant. You will have a baby that is like you and we don't want any more people like you.' "

A fourth area involves the notion that sex needs to be a secretive act. "Many individuals who were involved in relationships," Hingsburger notes about life in the institutions, "had never engaged in sexual intercourse in bed. Many had never even taken off all their clothing. Clients had learned to engage in institutional sex by standing up, where both parties need only pull up their pants and run if about to be discovered." As such, these individuals from the institutions do not understand that sexuality can be a good, healthy part of life.

Finally, many individuals may have had negative sexual experiences. "From being sexually abused as children or being punished for masturbation by parents," explains Hingsburger (1987), "to having all contacts with those of the opposite sex monitored and all discussion of sex forbidden, our clients have a broad range of negative experiences about sex and sexuality."

Individuals who had lived in institutions may present a more frightening story. Many clients who had lived in institutions had been molested as children or coerced into sexual activity within those institutions, and many of them had later become perpetrators of similar acts.

One worker describes the situation: "Characteristically, institutions — whether psychiatric or for the developmentally disabled — have been placed away from population centers, along with prisons. They also were in close proximity with military bases. Literally, some of the staff who worked in the institutions years ago would sell sexual favors to military personnel; they would be pimping out of the institutions. This kind of thing, thankfully, is not happening today. Honestly, I'm surprised that the people who did go through this system are able to function at all today."

Years ago, unfortunately, little attention had been focused on the problem of sexual exploitation of individuals with mental retardation (Haseltine and Miltenberger 1990), as revealed by the unavailability of statistics on the incidence of sexual abuse of clients on a national basis.

"The mentally retarded are vulnerable to sexual abuse," Haseltine et al. (1990) adds, "because of their dependence upon others for their basic needs, their compliance and passivity, their lack of social skills and judgment, and their lack of knowledge regarding basic preventative procedures."

Attitudes of Parents and Staff

While research suggests that mildly mentally retarded individuals are sexually expressive and capable of sexual discretion, they are often perceived as sexually incompetent. Concerning parents, research lists several instances (Abramson et al. 1988):

— Most parents of mentally retarded offspring fail to perceive their children as having sexual needs.

— In general, parents focus their concerns on inappropriate sexual expression and fears of exploitation.

— Many parents do not want their mentally retarded offspring to receive sex education, feeling that sex education will "overstimulate" their offspring's concern with sex.

Parents are not the only individuals who are discomforted by the sexual expression of mentally retarded people, however. Considerable distress is also evident among institutional and residential staff (Hall 1978 in Abramson et al. 1988). Parents, in comparison, often have less punitive and restrictive attitudes toward sexuality than do group home staff (McEwen 1977 in Pendler and Hingsburger 1990). Nonetheless, "as a consequence, and because sexually restrictive attitudes prevail among institutional staff mem-

182 | A GUIDE TO MENTAL RETARDATION

bers, many mentally retarded individuals are not permitted adequate sex lives" (Abramson et al. 1988).

Research

The research literature is filled with information which dispels most myths about the mentally retarded population. As Abramson et al. (1988) posits: "Sexual expression is significant to mentally retarded people. It is related to their personal happiness and enhances the stability of their intimate affiliations."

Studies have shown that sex education "does not fan the flames of wanton lust as previously believed, but quite to the contrary, increases adaptive behavior" (Coleman and Murphy 1980 in Hingsburger 1988). According to Edmonson, McCombs, and Wish (1979 in Hingsburger 1988), "I.Q. level is not a limitation on sexual knowledge. Moderately and severely handicapped individuals can acquire facts and attitudes that are components of self-sufficient and responsible behavior."

Addressing the belief that people who are mentally retarded possess inherently twisted sexual ideations, Edgerton (1973 in Abramson et al. 1988) explains that "sexual behavior of mentally retarded persons is learned, shaped, and reinforced by environmental factors. When in a community setting, their sexual behavior is similar to the sexual behavior of their same-age peers. Conversely, when mentally retarded individuals reside in an atypical environment, such as an institution, their sexual behavior is correspondingly atypical (that is, inappropriate masturbation, nonvolitional homosexuality, etc.)." Edgerton further contends that "mentally retarded individuals appear capable of stringent sexual self-control in both institutional and community settings; where, in both cases, sexual self-control was the product of internal regulation, not external constraint" (1973 in Abramson et al. 1988).

The General Lack of Meaningful Sex Education

For years parents and agencies have avoided the issue of sex education for persons with mental retardation due to conflicting emotions and moral beliefs (Hingsburger 1988). The extent, as described by Hingsburger and Griffiths (1986), has been to make sexuality a "nonissue" by establishing guidelines which state that

Adult Living | 183

"if clients wish to be sexual, they cannot receive residential services."

Some of these same attitudes continue today, and as a result many adults who live in the community do not possess the information and skills that would enable them to express their sexuality appropriately. When sexuality does become an issue, it usually takes the form of eliminating unwanted inappropriate sexual-type behaviors. Such behaviors may include inappropriate touching, grabbing or fondling of other peers, or various degrees of masturbatory behavior. These are behaviors which, for the most part, developed from life in the institutions or the lack of positive experiences. For some agencies, the focus may end there.

"What is dating to these people?" one worker asks. "To go out on a date . . . to have someone want to take you to a movie and buy you popcorn, to sit and put his arm around you. What is that? You may not be thinking that this person loves you, that he's only a friend. But many of these people are not aware of the consequences of dating, of the whole sexual activity that may be involved.

"That's a whole area that our agency realizes we have done little about. We've done Sexual Awareness Training, but that's it. We haven't taught that there are different kinds of love; that there are different kinds of feelings; that there are people who can be your friend, and it doesn't mean that you have to go to bed with them."

According to one researcher: "Mentally retarded individuals have rarely been provided with sex education programs. Perhaps as a consequence, many individuals incompletely evaluate the meaning and significance of dating, marriage, contraception, sexual intercourse, procreation, and abortion. The increased independence and patterns of social interaction now available to the retarded in the community necessitate that this issue no longer be ignored" (Sengstock 1972 in Abramson et al. 1988).

Fortunately, attitudes are changing, if slowly: "Parents, public school systems, group homes, and training programs are beginning to provide the mentally retarded with sex education" (Sengstock 1972 in Abramson et al. 1988). Furthermore, research indicates that sex education "greatly increases contraceptive, reproductive, and hygienic knowledge; improves social skills; and reduces inappropriate behavior of mentally retarded people"

184 | A GUIDE TO MENTAL RETARDATION

(Demetral 1981 in Abramson et al. 1988). "To be effective with this population, sex education curricula must be specially designed" (Abramson et al. 1988).

When provided with the proper sex education that meets the individual's needs, persons with mental retardation show improvements in adaptive behavior (Coleman and Murphy 1980 in Hingsburger 1988). For example, Foxx, McMorro, Storey, and Rogers (1984), after implementing a social/sexual training program for institutionalized adults with mental retardation, found that their subjects' appropriate social responses to sexually related situations increased during training and generalized to other situations beyond their training program.

Considering the question of whether persons who are mentally retarded are capable of conscientious contraception, Hall (1975 in Abramson et al. 1988) presents that mildly mentally retarded women were capable of successfully managing contraceptive pills.

Haseltine et al. (1990), having developed a curriculum for teaching self-protection skills to mentally retarded adults — teaching them to say "No," to leave the situation, and to report an inappropriate incident — find that seven out of eight students learned and maintained such skills for at least six months and were able to generalize these skills to other settings.

Education and support have been geared toward parents and helping staff as well. Pendler and Hingsburger (1990), having developed a group approach to working with parents, offer a glimpse of hope: "The excitement of running a parental group to discuss sexuality and sex education is that these topics go far beyond biology to the broader view of the developmentally handicapped as *full adults*. Parents have to come to the realization that their children may have the potential for full, productive, and loving lives" (emphasis added).

Sexual Awareness Training

Training in sexual awareness has been instituted in one agency only as recently as five years ago. According to the current coordinator of their Sexual Awareness Training Program, "The main thrust of our efforts is to try to ensure that the clients have their rights protected, and that staff do their part as providers to protect the clients.

Adult Living | 185

"We have a system in place now which I have been coordinating for about five years. We run groups using a format developed by the Letchworth Village Social Work department several years ago — lesson plans and things like that — to help clients learn about sexuality. But not just sexuality: they learn how to relate to others; how they are different from and the same as other people; notions of social responsibility, and so on.

"The program begins by asking: 'How are you the same and how are you different?' We begin with the real basics in terms of self-identification, regardless of gender; the basic physical characteristics of the person, which is the way most people begin to understand similarities and differences.

"The program then progresses from 'self' and how you're the same and yet different from others — which is self-awareness — to group awareness, in terms of how you conduct yourself within a group and how group members can be different. From here, we move into general social awareness in terms of expectations of the community, and so on. For example, to teach that we would not go into a public place and do certain kinds of things that we would do in private.

"After several sessions we get into the area which may be recognized as sexually charged material. But there's a whole range of social consciousness raising that goes on in the groups prior to getting into sexual areas. Ultimately, once it does get involved, the program talks about responsibility of sexually active individuals in terms of contraception and preventing sexually transmitted diseases (STD). Obviously, we talk a lot about the use of a condom as a pivotal point in the program; that a condom should be used when engaging in certain types of sexual contact. Also, we counsel that, under no circumstances in our society, is the notion of rape acceptable; they need to understand that coercion is not something that is acceptable.

"The groups have worked fairly well. Once a person goes through the system — the group itself — what they have learned, in terms of education and health and safety issues, will be presented to their Interdisciplinary Treatment Team (ITT). The team will then make a decision as to whether the individual has learned enough in the program to protect themselves, to protect others, and to act as responsibly as possible regarding sexual expression with another person. In this case, the team may say, 'We think this

186 | A GUIDE TO MENTAL RETARDATION

person has learned enough to engage in sex with another person who has gone through the program.'

"Both parties, if they live in a residence, will have to have gone through the program — not the entire program, necessarily, but gone through enough of it. In some cases, when individuals refuse this program, we can have some work done by outside organizations such as Planned Parenthood, if that is more comfortable for the individuals. Frankly, this is indicated, since as an agency we try to get people linked with community services in the first place.

"At whatever stage the individual's treatment team feels the individual understands the competency and health-and-safety issues, the agency can allow the expression of sexuality with another individual who has a similar competency.

"It doesn't have to come from the sexuality program, per se. Certainly, people start at very different levels. They don't have to go through the whole program; they would just have to have covered the basics.

"For people who live in our residential programs and have relationships outside of the residential program, it is obvious that we can't expect the person on the outside to be similarly trained. What we do hope is that the information we have given to the people in our program will be used outside the program as well.

"And so, basically, we have to try and preserve the rights of the individuals that we serve, but balance that with our responsibilities as caregivers to protect them. This, characteristically, is where we run into conflict in the system.

"We have to understand — based upon some of the statistics from the Adult Protective Services and Child Protective Services — that, of the people with whom we work, probably ninety-nine percent or more, if they have been institutionalized, they have been sexually molested or sexually abused at some point in their history.

"These are the sort of people with whom we are starting to work. And it is difficult to teach people who came from a system that told them that sex was not for them, that they shouldn't get involved, that they're not competent. Now they are trying to unlearn all of that, and we are trying to help them to understand that they can talk about feelings and issues in a safe way." (Note: An excellent source for dealing with sex counseling with the developmentally handicapped can be found in Hingsburger 1987.)

Dealing with Denial

"There's a lot of denial when you come from an environment that says that sex is not for you as a person because you're just not up to it. You wind up denying a lot of your feelings. I'm sure there's a great deal of stimulation regarding feelings; that many of these feelings that are not dealt with openly are going to be turned into other kinds of behavior.

"I think that we see some behaviors based on the fact that people are frustrated regarding their ability to express and engage in what meets basic human needs. We're trying to undo that now, but it takes quite a bit of time to accomplish this."

Marriage and Parenthood

Marriage

Many individuals with mental retardation view marriage as an important role in life — a symbol of acceptance and normalcy and a needed means of belonging and sharing. The issues of marriage and parenthood are closely allied with sexuality, and elicit similar concerns from the community regarding the rights of adults with mental retardation (Patton et al. 1986). Yet the laws within many states still restrict and prohibit marriage between "feebleminded" persons (Patton et al. 1986).

But based upon various research, a different picture emerges. Research reports the following:

— Marriage among persons with mild retardation is only slightly below the national average (Ingalls 1978 in Patton et al. 1986).

— Women with mental retardation marry more frequently than do men with mental retardation.

— Persons with mental retardation possess the capacity and desire for successful marriages, as research suggests that mildly

188 | A GUIDE TO MENTAL RETARDATION

retarded individuals are capable of maintaining happy and stable marriages with other retarded and nonretarded persons (Craft and Craft 1979 in Abramson et al. 1988).

— When accompanied by financial and emotional support, such marriages have a high likelihood for success (Hall 1975 in Abramson et al. 1988).

"With appropriate preparation, training, and continued understanding and help," one author strongly contends, "mildly retarded adults . . . make as good a marital adjustment as nonretarded persons in the same socioeconomic circumstances" (Katz 1972 in Patton et al. 1986).

Parenthood

Of all issues regarding people who have mental retardation, parenthood stirs the hottest fears and debates. "Society, at large," one worker explains, "has a difficult time accepting that individuals who are mentally retarded can have normal children. In addition, there is a valid concern as to the life of a child who might be born to parents who are developmentally disabled."

Is this fear valid? As one worker reveals, "I think this is an admirable concern of society. I believe that everyone in society would want to see a child get the best shot at growing up and making it on his own at some point."

Nonetheless, the facts are surprising:

— Persons with mental retardation have a lower rate of reproduction — perhaps are less fertile — than individuals without retardation (Craft and Craft 1979 in Abramson et al. 1988).

— Parents with mental retardation run a higher risk of producing offspring with mental retardation. The chance of producing offspring with mental retardation is 40% when both parents have mental retardation, 15% when one parent has mental retardation, and only 1% when neither parent has mental retardation (Reed and Reed 1965, Hall 1975 in Abramson et al. 1988).

But are married adults who are disabled able to provide adequate parenting? Research in this area has been problematic (Tymchuck, Andron, and Unger 1987 in Abramson et al. 1988). Some studies, for instance, report that approximately 15% of mentally retarded parents have their children removed from the home; however, it is unknown whether this reflects inadequate

Adult Living | 189

childcare, unacceptable variation in parenting style, economic limits, or ineffective presentation and representation in courts (Craft and Craft 1981 in Abramson et al. 1988).

"There is a great deal of support out in the community for children of developmentally disabled parents and the parents themselves," one worker tells. "I think as the view of society changes, there will be more support to keep the child's needs met while staying with the parents — needs other than emotional needs, which disabled parents already meet fairly well."

Summary

While issues of human rights, legal protection, and quality of life remain vitally important *throughout* the lives of individuals with mental retardation, adulthood introduces new issues. Specialized training programs are designed to enable individuals to demonstrate competence as adults in the community by emphasizing social skills as well as job skills. And legal advocacy and protection agencies,m are able to intervene whenever there is a question about the infringement of a client's constitutional or civil rights.

Yet, while progress is being made in the system, historically the general population has had many misconceptions about people who have mental retardation. Misconceptions about the social issues around the sexuality of adults with mental retardation are still being addressed and challenged, and professionals in the field are working toward improving education — current and appropriate sexual awareness training is now being offered to adults with mental retardation. But equally important, there needs to be education of the general population to avoid repeating mistakes of the past, and to allow adults with mental retardation to have full lives — lives which can include marriage and parenthood.

6

Senior Living

Need for Development and Innovation

Mental retardation is the single largest category of lifelong handicaps (Seltzer and Krauss 1987). Ironically, professionals in the field have spent decades focused almost exclusively on the care and understanding of children with disabilities (Seltzer and Krauss 1987). That may be one reason persons with mental retardation have been viewed as children, and often treated like them, even in adulthood (Seltzer and Krauss 1987). Only in the early 1970s did adults with mental retardation begin to receive a substantial amount of focus and concern, drawing attention to the need for age-appropriate services.

Until recently, the range of services which have addressed the needs of adults with mental retardation did not include any consideration of the needs of elderly persons with mental retardation (Seltzer and Krauss 1987). The pattern of research and service development is best illustrated by Seltzer and Krauss (1987): "It is not surprising that fifteen years after the time when the field expanded its vision to include adulthood, we are now straining our eyes to examine the next stage, namely old age."

192 | A GUIDE TO MENTAL RETARDATION

Factors Influencing Service Systems and Policy-Makers

Increased Population

Elderly persons with mental retardation currently are receiving a somewhat privileged status among policy-makers, planners, and researchers who are acknowledging, somewhat belatedly, that the number of persons with mental retardation aged fifty-five or over is large and that the numbers are growing (Kavanagh 1988). Experts in the field say there are now at least 200,000 people with mental retardation over sixty years of age in the United States (*The New York Times*, October 28, 1990).

Estimates of the number of elderly persons with mental retardation are needed for long-range planning. However, as Seltzer and Krauss point out, "It may be invalid to use estimates based on the number of known service recipients for future planning purposes because many persons who are mentally retarded and over age fifty-five are not currently known to the formal service system." It is estimated that only about 40% of the estimated number of elderly persons with mental retardation are known to the formal service system (Krauss 1986 in Seltzer et al. 1987).

Increased Longevity

The advances in longevity have been especially dramatic for those individuals with Down syndrome, the leading known cause for mental retardation (*The New York Times*, October 28, 1990). In the 1940s, Down syndrome babies had a life expectancy of only twelve years. Today, most are living well into their fifties (*The New York Times*, October 28, 1990). Most people with other forms of mental retardation, except those so profoundly retarded that they cannot walk or feed themselves, now live close to normal life spans (*The New York Times*, October 28, 1990), where an estimated 50% of people with retardation now live beyond age fifty-five (Richards and Siddiqui 1980 in Barcikowska et al. 1989).

Increased Vulnerability

As with any elderly population, longer life brings with it an increased vulnerability to chronic illness and disability (Seltzer et al.

1987). Therefore, special medical attention is due the elderly mentally retarded individual as with any medically fragile senior.

Decreasing Support Systems

According to Seltzer et al. (1987), there are proportionately fewer younger people to provide support for the elderly mentally retarded population who are in need of care.

Some Characteristics
of Elderly Persons with Mental Retardation

Adaptive Functioning and Health

It is generally assumed that older persons with mental retardation have more health problems and limitations than younger adults. However, while some research provides support for this assumption, others do not (Seltzer and Krauss 1987).

While one group of researchers found that elderly persons with mental retardation received more medical services than younger adults in the sample, suggesting that the seniors had more serious medical needs (Janicki and MacEachron 1984 in Seltzer et al. 1987), other studies found that elderly and younger adult sample members did not differ in the number of health problems (Seltzer, Seltzer, and Sherwood 1982 in Seltzer and Krauss 1987). Furthermore, while it is reported that elderly persons with mental retardation were more functionally impaired than the younger group studied (Seltzer at al. 1982 in Seltzer and Krauss 1987), other researchers found that, with important exceptions for particular subgroups, "Older persons with mental retardation function at a significantly higher level than their younger counterparts" (Krauss and Seltzer 1986 in Kavanagh 1988).

One worker, recalling an article concluding that the level of overall deterioration — mental and physical — for developmentally disabled people was actually less than the deterioration rate among the general population throughout the aging process, provides the following explanation: "I think part of the reason is people who are developmentally delayed are not as stressed by aging and the limitations that it brings them because they are more matter-of-fact about themselves and their lives. They have been allowed to do less, so the limitations don't change their life dramatically. Whereas a person who is aging in the normal population, losing their ability to make choices and be self-sustaining, the impact of that is very stressful and filled with emotional reactions."

A worker who has much exposure to seniors with mental retardation recalls one example: "One woman had a radical mastectomy. Her reaction was 'Oh, it was sore, but I'm better now.' She certainly was as traumatized as anyone would be by that kind of surgery. But her thought processes are far less involved: she may not be as concerned with the loss of a breast or the larger implications of having cancer."

One reason for such disparity in research findings on seniors has been posited by Seltzer and Krauss (1987) who offer two possible explanations. "First, the elderly individual may seem less seriously retarded than their younger counterparts because the elderly include 'borderline' persons with mental retardation who, today, would not be labeled mentally retarded and who are thus not included statistically with a younger population. Second, the younger population receiving services includes a disproportionate number of severely and profoundly retarded person who are unlikely to live to old age."

National Distribution of Programs for Elderly Persons with Mental Retardation

There is a great deal of disparity among states in the number of programs for elderly persons with mental retardation that have been developed. Given the current stage of program development for elderly persons, this is not surprising. As described by Seltzer and Krauss (1987), "The development of programs for elderly persons with mental retardation began largely as a grassroots movement in response to needs identified by operators of programs for retarded adults approaching old age, by families of aging retarded persons, and by advocacy organizations."

Based upon a national survey of existing programs for elderly persons with mental retardation, Seltzer and Krauss (1987) report that, of those locations taking part of the survey, there exist 327 community-based facilities and 202 which were institutionally based. However, while the number of programs for elderly persons with mental retardation is not large nationally, the programs tend to be clustered geographically.

For example, all but seven states had at least one program for the elderly mentally retarded population. New York State has the largest number of programs, either institution- or community-based, with 113 locations. following by Massachusetts with 54 programs, California with 31 programs, and Pennsylvania with 30 programs (Seltzer and Krauss 1987).

One could argue that this cluster in available programming is not necessarily a negative indication of future directions. As Seltzer and Krauss (1987) summarize, "There is reason for optimism in the continued growth of programs serving elderly mentally retarded persons. First, it is a national phenomenon. Second, programs are developing . . . at a more rapid rate than ever before reported."

Present Service Options

Concerns about the needs of persons with mental retardation as they age and the capacities of existing service systems to meet those needs have been expressed since the early 1960s into the 1970s. However, guidelines are needed to help develop or restructure programs to meet the varied needs of older and elderly persons with mental retardation and have only recently begun to appear (Seltzer and Krauss 1987).

(1) Age Integration Option

The most common approach to providing services to elderly persons with mental retardation is to include them in programs now serving mentally retarded adults of all ages (Seltzer and Krauss 1987). There is evidence which suggests that elderly mentally retarded service recipients, as a group, do not necessarily function at a lower level than younger persons with mental retardation (Janicki and MacEachron 1984 in Seltzer and Krauss 1987). As a

196 | A GUIDE TO MENTAL RETARDATION

result, maintaining or integrating some aging persons with mental retardation into programs for younger adults with mental retardation, without dramatically modifying the services offered, is viewed as a viable alternative.

(2) Specialized Service Option

The specialized service option is capturing considerable attention among researchers, planners, and program developers. Within this option, special services are developed for elderly persons with mental retardation in order to respond to their special needs (Seltzer and Krauss 1987). Program features within this option include slower paced programming, more opportunities for personal choice, more recreational and leisure time activities, and increased attention to health needs of elderly persons with mental retardation (Seltzer and Krauss 1987).

(3) Generic Services Option

The generic services option integrates persons with mental retardation into services designed for the general, nonretarded, elderly population. Interestingly, this is the least common option in day programming for elderly persons with mental retardation, but the most common option for residential programs (Seltzer and Krauss 1987).

The advantages of this option are best illustrated by Seltzer and Krauss (1987): "High-functioning elderly mentally retarded persons may be excellent candidates for mainstreaming into generic senior citizen programs, as they generally compare favorably with nonretarded elderly persons who, themselves, may have serious chronic illnesses and cognitive functional limitations," further adding that "the diagnosis of mental retardation alone should not be seen as a barrier to utilization of generic services." However, while there are generic senior citizen programs that accept persons with mental retardation, and indeed have positive experiences to report (Seltzer and Krauss 1987), the absolute number of persons with mental retardation involved in such programs nationwide is estimated to be very small (Seltzer and Krauss 1987).

Senior Living | 197

Similar Characteristics of Aging Populations in General

"From the seminars that I've been involved with in the past couple of years," one active worker discusses, "it seems that there is a lot of push in this state and other states to integrate services for the aging population overall. I think people realize that the characteristics of any aging population tend to converge as their age increases — the disabled population and so-called normal population begin to converge in terms of their limitations and their problems, medical issues, loss of mental capacity. There are a lot of similarities.

"I know from seeing an Alzheimer's group that those people, in general, have lower functioning and need more hand-over-hand, one-on-one intervention than most developmentally disabled seniors. You'll see both groups with individuals who are nonverbal or withdrawn. You look at some retarded people — they repeat and repeat; and then you look at a lot of older people — they repeat and repeat."

As both populations show similar characteristics, more efficient use of funding is possible. "People are becoming aware that you really can do a lot more with the money that's available rather than have two separate programs," one worker suggests. "Particularly if you have a population with similar characteristics, especially in light of what seems to be a relative increase in Alzheimer's among aging people. A lot of money would be saved if we brought people together; there would be twice as much money to deal with the problem and develop programs."

Benefits of Integration

"There is a big push to integrate elderly people of the general population into adult day-care senior centers so they can have relationships with their peers," presents one worker. "I know a program where the people come to the senior day-care or senior center looking for things to do. When they become involved with the population of developmentally disabled individuals, they have a sense of fulfillment because they are in a helping position. They also have this peer relationship with people that they've never really met before; I think they are less defensive at that point in their lives and they are less judgmental of those people, and it gives them a sense of fulfillment to interact with them — not necessarily just in a helping capacity, but just having the opportunity to interact."

There are a number of examples of an integrated environment existing in the community. A worker describes one of them: "We are registered as part of the Retired Senior Volunteer Program (RSVP), which is a county program. At this point, we have only done volunteer work. We are set up to be involved with the county infirmary, to fold clothes for their laundry, to feed people at the nursing home. When I get a chance to go to the Office of the Aging, I will find out what is available. And then, slowly, we can have visits, luncheons, etc., and see what happens."

Can integration happen without resistance? "I don't think you can totally break down the barriers immediately. You have the same obstacles that you faced when you opened up a community house or whenever you try to integrate a population into a normalized setting. The staff of a senior center may be a little worried about being around mentally retarded people. They may wonder: 'Are they going to hurt someone? How are our seniors going to react?'

"Again, the normal senior population may have their own prejudices to deal with. They may say, 'That person is retarded. Don't put him near me.'

"I think it has to be a very gradual process. First, you have to get the staff engaged in dialogue."

Future Directions

Research, primarily, involves those elderly persons with mental retardation receiving services. However, evidence suggests that there are an equal number of elderly persons with mental retardation who are not known to the service network (Seltzer and Krauss 1987). These "unknown" people may be living independently with no formal contact with services, living with family members, or living in residential settings outside the scope of a service system (Kavanagh 1988). Obviously, much needs to be learned about this population to aid in developing sound, long-term care policies (Seltzer 1985 in Kavanagh 1988).

The following is taken from an interview with a mental retardation professional actively involved in a seniors committee connected with a local ARC, and a member of the Task Force for Aging Services.

Q: Describe your involvement with the aging population of persons with mental retardation.

Basically, [we have a] Seniors Committee to direct some of the senior services that are going to be offered by the agency over the next few years. The committee is very much in its infancy, but meets frequently to look at different aspects of what is happening in the field of aging mentally retarded people.

I am also involved in a ten-county Task Force for Aging Services. It has been the trend to create these task force enclaves around the state to generate demographics and program options for our area. . . .

Under the Task Force committee, there are two other subcommittees. One is trying to publish guidelines for senior programs — a kind of generic manual of considerations for any agency getting into aging services. The other is a Training and Technical Assistance committee, which will go through the ten-county area and use the guidelines manual as a tool to sensitize staff and agencies as to what they should be planning for their aging people.

Q: What are some issues dealt with by the Task Force for Aging Services?

There are basically two sides to what is going on. First, you have people who have lived in institutions for forty, fifty, even sixty years who, because the institutions are closing, are now being placed in community settings. As a result, these people are feeling like they have lost their families and their homes because they think of the staff and the institution as their home. They are being placed in community settings without being given a choice.

Furthermore, they are being forced to participate in "active treatment programs." Some of them are very excited about this because they want to work, while others are very resentful because

200 | A GUIDE TO MENTAL RETARDATION

they feel uprooted. They may feel: "Why do I have to move? I don't want to do this. Why should I have to do it now? I am eighty years old; leave me alone!" They are being placed in settings like ICFs and CRs, day programs, and workshops. It's kind of like a double-edged sword: you have both worlds that you have to consider.

On the other hand, you have people who have lived in residential settings during their twenties, thirties, and forties, have worked for years, and are now facing retirement. They want to be able to retire from workshop settings, but still receive some type of pension like "normal" people do. They want to stay in their residential settings even though their medical needs may be requiring attention. If they are in a supervised setting they may require a little bit more medical attention due to their natural aging process, or they may require more time off. They may want to be able to nap in the afternoon but then go back to work.

There are a lot of issues that are being dealt with state-side by a lot of these isolated task forces around the state. Working area by area, these task forces are trying to come up with model programs. . . .

There are a lot of unique things happening in the field, but we feel like we are at the beginning, just prodding along a step at a time to try to compensate for everyone.

Q: What is the trend, or future direction, for aging services?

The trend is really very much to integrate, as much as possible, geriatric populations with aging persons with mental retardation.

We have found that mental retardation was basically labeled back around the turn of the century for various reasons that have nothing to do with mental retardation. Historically, mental retardation was an umbrella that encompassed physical deformity, a family not able to cope with mental illness, or a lot of other reasons. This institutionalization led to different categories of disability over time. There is no one answer to mental retardation and I don't think there is going to be for a long period of time.

Q: Will senior populations served in these agencies be more homogeneous in the future?

Ideally, yes. It would be really nice to see it happen because what we are finding now is that there is very little difference in the needs between our seniors here who have been through lifelong institutionalization and those generic seniors living in a senior residence. For a generic senior — a nonhandicapped senior perhaps eighty years old who has lost [his or her] house for financial reasons and is no longer working — the needs are identical. They get together in a room and you have no idea who came from what social system.

Q: Describe the distinction with the Down syndrome aging population and how seniors agencies address this issue.

Basically, we have in this facility of twenty-six people all three worlds. We have the person who was institutionalized at the turn of the century because of physical deformities who [wasn't] necessarily mentally retarded when they were two or three years old. Now they are seventy and want to work for the first time in their lives. Then we have people who would be like our parents, who would just go on and retire.

Then there are groups of people who have needs in terms of their bodies aging more quickly than their chronological age. Someone with Down syndrome may be sixty, but yet their body may appear to be ninety. They need a slower paced day; they need more frequent naps; they need more frequent medical care. Someone with a degenerative bone condition or degenerative arthritis would fit into that same category. Their needs are very similar in terms of medical supervision and prevention of rapid regression and loss of skills that have been learned in their life time.

Q: How does your senior center stand in relation to the programs developed for the population of mentally retarded seniors in New York State?

When the building first opened six years ago, it was a one-of-a-kind proposal. One, because of its size. Usually, residences were ten or twelve beds, which is becoming the trend again, so there will not be a place this size again.

202 | A GUIDE TO MENTAL RETARDATION

Q: What were some of the problems faced because of the size of this facility?

Number one, when we first opened, all twenty-six people were to attend in-house day programming. With all of the preparations that have to go into opening a new facility with state numbers and social service numbers, it turned out that a lot of people were misplaced. There was no way that you could expect twenty-six people who were not necessarily medically fragile to stay in this building all of the time and have a certified program.

Q: In other words, a smaller number of residents is ideal, although having a day treatment program connected to this senior residence is a good idea as well?

Yes. That is truly what made this center unique. We are more functional for medically frail people — people that require a longer rest period after lunch, or after dinner, or a later sleep-in time in the morning. It's not necessary for them to get up and go out to the vans every morning to drive into town. Sometimes these van trips could be an hour long.

Q: What are some other advantages of this kind of model seniors program?

We have the advantage of having a flexible day program. Currently, under the new "active treatment regulations," anything can be called active treatment. Now, we can go out on trips with small groups of people.

Frequently, persons at a formalized day program, because of the sizes of programs and different classrooms, get "locked" into that routine. They can't take trips as easily as we can here. There are so many different varieties of things we can do, such as baking classes.

Q: Will senior centers be categorized?

We are in the situation where we can't be categorized. However, that is the trend for all facilities that are being opened . . . just to be homogeneous according to whatever their population is and to be totally needs-driven so that you are not calling yourself an ICF or a nursing home or anything like that. Instead, you are calling yourself a facility that is going to meet the needs of the people who live in it, which is exactly what this center does.

This definitely is the way everything is going. They are not going to categorize and label. I think for seniors it is going to be much easier to do, just because of the size of the population that is coming out of the nursing homes and the large numbers of people within agencies who are reaching fifty-five and above; the agencies don't know what to do anymore. There are a large number of people who are getting up in age who are not going to be able to stay in the workshops much longer because of staffing ratio and for safety reasons.

Q: How is staffing here different than at other programs?

For most of the other ICFs, all of the people leave the house for their day program, so the houses are basically empty during the day except for housekeeping and administrative staff.

Here, we have fifteen people — a full clinical team — present at day programming. And because programming is very flexible, there may be four people out with one staff member at the mall getting their hair cut or shopping, two other people out with the nurses on an appointment, and six left in the day program doing class work (which most institutionalized people look forward to Monday through Friday). We can also compensate for someone who needs to convalesce from a hospital stay. We have nurses here that are on call twenty-four hours a day, in addition to a medical director who is on call whenever we need his services. There is a lot more flexibility. It is basically a medical model with the social model added in. Our clients are here basically because of their medical needs.

Q: The ICF is a medical model in theory, designed to get a person coming out of institutions healthy in order to move on to a less restrictive environment. How is your program viewed along these lines?

204 | A GUIDE TO MENTAL RETARDATION

We can't really be designated as a true ICF. So we are called a Geriatric ICF, to set us apart a little bit from the rest of the ICF program — because of the in-house day program, because of the need for a flexible day program. There are a lot of clients here who take a nap after lunch. That isn't typical in a day treatment setting.

When someone here is seriously ill you sometimes see other residents taking care of that one person — getting staff, saying "So-and-so is having trouble sleeping." It is very much like its own unique community.

Q: Are the demands placed on staff here any different than other residential placements?

Yes. Because of the diversity of the people who are here — we have some people who are profoundly retarded and therefore cannot control their verbal outbursts — it is hard to explain something like this to someone who is ninety who just wants a quiet place to sit. We also have some people who are mentally ill *and* have behavior problems, which can pose a physical threat to someone who is medically frail.

There is a real need for more medically and behaviorally trained staff; the demand on staff here is greater than in any other ICF or day program. For example, I think the lowest number of medications we have ever passed out in one day was sixty-six. Staff are required by auditors to be knowledgeable about all those medications. Staff need to be aware of the side effects. They are also required to provide a lot of first aid care, medical care, prevention of skin breakdown and bed sores for people who may be bed-bound; there are many people here who are physically involved that need to be lifted. And then we have a behavioral component, where we want to protect the medically frail people from someone else's aggressive behaviors.

Q: Working with aging persons with mental retardation, as with any frail elderly person in a nursing home, must be difficult due to the number of deaths involved and the need to deal with this issue for this population.

It is hard to keep staff motivated and not apathetic. We have had five deaths in the past year alone, which was a lot for us. Before that, we had only one or two deaths a year; the medical director kept telling us, "You should expect at least four deaths a year," and we said, "Nah." Well, he taught us a lesson this past year because we had five and it was difficult.

It was especially difficult because we are dealing with staff's feelings as well as those of the residents.A lot of times, we found, over the past year in particular, that the people who lived here handled the situation a lot better than staff did. The residents were supporting the staff, rather than the other way around, which is unique.

I think this has helped us grow up a bit, as well as influence the direction that this place is going. It is being run much more by the people who live here than by the people who work here. It is something that we have tried to do subtly, but is coming of its own making, which is nice to see.

Q: Why do you think they had been better able to deal with the death of friends or acquaintances?

They are much more accustomed to change. They were the people who were yanked out of the institutions and told, "You are going to live someplace else," and put there. They are the people who see their peers getting ill and then getting healthy again.

They are much more society-wise than we are. We usually have our small circle of family and very close friends. They have seen people walk in and out of their lives so much. This is especially true for people who are really physically handicapped, who require staff to help them toilet and bathe and meet their personal hygiene needs — needs met all their lives by people who have abused them over so many years in their previous placements. They are simply much more adaptable than we ever give them credit [for being].

Some individuals are not as adaptable, however. There are those choice few who, whenever a change occurs, resent it and continue to resent it for the rest of their lives. The way that they show this resentment is through behavioral outbursts or manipula-

206 | A GUIDE TO MENTAL RETARDATION

tive behavior. Even this, to a certain extent, is understandable; they are taking control.

Q: Where does the program currently stand in state-wide development of services for elderly persons with developmental disabilities?

It is really hard to say. I think the program has reached a plateau with all the changes in the agency. We are no longer at the forefront of facilities in the state offering really quality senior programs. There are a couple of other programs around that are unique in their offerings; some of the programs have been offered grants for integrating senior centers and OMRDD programs.

Q: How are these other facilities more creative?

These programs take into consideration ideas from the guidelines for seniors programs we just finished writing. An example would involve environmental factors, such as not having the wall the same color as the floor like we do in our building. When people start to age, their eyesight goes and their perceptual skills are different. Therefore, you need rooms that are brighter in color.

There is a lot more awareness of the general geriatric person now, and there is also more knowledge about OMRDD geriatric people that is starting to surface. The university [here] is in partnership with a coalition in [the city] for an aging task force, and they are offering programs in gerontology and developmental disabilities. With this increase in knowledge and understanding, people will no longer be saying, "Well, that's the way retarded people are going to look past age sixty." There are more options becoming available to everyone at the same time.

I think we could be a lot more creative than is currently the case. However, being the agency that we are, we are trying to cover the entire life span of a person throughout our various programs — a balancing act at best.

Working with Family Members

"Many parents of offspring with mental retardation never expect to face the worry of who will take care of their son or daughter if something should happen to themselves. However, unlike most of their peers born over a generation ago, persons with mental retardation today may begin to outlive their parents. In many cases, because of improved living conditions and medical advances, they will reach their own old age" (Kavanagh 1988).

As a result, parents are now facing difficult decisions about whether to place their offspring in a group home, or to ask sons or daughters to take responsibility for their sibling with mental retardation (*The New York Times,* October 28, 1990). Most mothers who have cared for their children at home feel that no one else will care as well.

Parents who have taken care of their retarded children for so many years want some kind of fictional resolution in which, minutes before the parent dies, the child dies of some natural cause. The parent cannot imagine their offspring being able to go on and be well cared for after they are dead (Kavanagh 1988).

One of the devices that has been successfully used is to offer some legal service, for example, estate planning and will writing, which often helps the family begin to think and talk about issues involved with death and dying, their own and that of the retarded family member (Kavanagh 1988).

Support Systems

Since the majority of persons with mental retardation at any age do not live in public or private residential settings, it is inferred that the number of aging persons with mental retardation is considerable, although many of these persons are not currently in contact with the formal service system (Seltzer 1985). However, little is known about the pattern of family relationships and supports for elderly persons with mental retardation. It can be assumed, however, from past research on the general population "that maintenance of some contact with family members is very important with respect to the quality of life for aging persons with mental retardation" (Seltzer and Krauss 1987).

The value of informal support systems for the aging person with mental retardation, as for the general aging population, is great. Informal support systems reduce the impact of declining functional abilities, helps elderly persons maintain their lifestyles,

208 | A GUIDE TO MENTAL RETARDATION

limits the adverse effects associated with bereavement, supports a higher rate of participation in social activities, and is associated with lower rates of depression and utilization of formal services (Seltzer 1985). Furthermore, there is strong evidence that a major antecedent of institutionalization among nonretarded elderly persons is the absence of informal supports (Seltzer 1985), although valid generalization to the mentally retarded population remains unknown.

Informal Supports

In the general population, it is the formal support system — primarily the family — that provides the bulk of services for elderly persons; in most cases, support is provided by a spouse or by daughters, daughters-in-law, or sons (Seltzer 1985). Unlike most in the elderly population, however, aging persons with mental retardation generally do not have children or a spouse on whom they can depend for support. In some cases, there are very old parents who still provide some support to the already elderly retarded person (Seltzer 1985).

In most cases, the family network for individuals with mental retardation consists of brothers and sisters, and possibly the children of their brothers and sisters (Seltzer 1985). Based upon a study of 450 families, 80% of the adults with retardation who have siblings get at least some help from them. Furthermore, about 60% of the families said that a brother or sister would supervise their sibling's care if the parents were no longer able (*The New York Times,* October 28, 1990).

For the general population, sibling relationships are typically of the longest duration of any human relationship, and possibly the most equal of all those within the family (Seltzer 1985). "I've seen families where the siblings are very involved and act as backup," one worker shares. "When the parents are deceased, siblings take someone in, or act as that person's primary contact, and keep a close family contact. Sometimes, many siblings will do this."

When one sibling is retarded, however, "the egalitarian quality of the sibling relationship is compromised to some degree" (Seltzer 1985). While long-term relationships between elderly persons with mental retardation and their siblings is relatively unknown (Seltzer 1985), an important issue in need of research is the extent to which aging siblings maintain relationships and provide support to their also-aging retarded family members (Seltzer 1985).

It is possible that the role of friends might be even more important for elderly persons with mental retardation, given their more limited circle of relatives at this time in life (Seltzer 1985). The extent to which aging retarded persons exchange informal support with their friends is unknown (Seltzer 1985); however, it is likely that at the least, emotional support is gained from these relationships (O'Connor 1983 in Seltzer 1985).

Aiding in the development and maintenance of these friendships, no less, is an important consideration for aging persons with mental retardation. Unfortunately, as a result of moving retarded adults from setting to setting as their level of functioning changes, these friendships don't always have a chance to survive. As one author notes: "We move them away from those settings where their friends work and live, in spite of the fact that we have learned that their social interactions are far more important to many of them than our middle-class work ethic" (O'Connor 1983 in Seltzer 1985).

Remaining Home

Studies have shown that elderly retarded persons have only limited contact with their families (Seltzer 1985), and very few are known to live with their relatives (Seltzer 1985). Based upon various researchers, over half (52.2%) of the approximately 59,000 persons with mental retardation receiving some services live in their natural family home (Meyers, Borthwick, and Eyman 1985 in Kavanagh 1988). Once the person with mental retardation reaches age fifty-five, however, about 25% of all persons with mild retardation, 20% of persons with moderate retardation, 8% of persons with severe retardation, and about 3% of persons with profound retardation still live with their natural families (Meyers et al. 1985 in Kavanagh 1988).

"Although it may be difficult to many families to make it possible for an elderly retarded relative to live in their house-

210 | A GUIDE TO MENTAL RETARDATION

hold," Seltzer (1985) comments, "the maintenance of some contact with family members is undoubtedly very important with respect to the quality of life of aging retarded persons."

Stressors on Informal Supports

While informal supports for elderly persons with mental retardation is important, there are a number of factors that limit the availability of informal support systems.

Various factors have been illustrated (Hooyman 1983 in Seltzer 1985). First, families are having fewer children, so fewer family members exist to care for the person with mental retardation as he ages.

Second, divorce rates are increasing, and when the nuclear family is disrupted it can limit its ability to care for the elderly relative with mental retardation. Third, as families become more mobile geographically, the proximity of potential helpers decreases.

Finally, as more and more women become increasingly involved in the work force, their availability to provide care for their elderly retarded relatives decreases.

Finding a Specialized Group Home

"Facilities are seeing a lot more two-generation geriatric families, with a very old parent and a retarded child who is old himself. Families are sometimes on a waiting list for more than ten years" for services (*The New York Times,* October 28, 1990).

Presented here are descriptions and comparisons of general programs for elderly persons with mental retardation based upon a national survey conducted by Seltzer and Krauss (1987).

Community-Based Residential Programs

Group Homes

In general, group homes are professionally staffed residences for persons with disabilities. They provide an individual with training in daily living activities, opportunities for recreation, and a supportive environment for the development of skills for increased independence (Seltzer and Krauss 1987).

When compared to alternative placements, group homes are the most common form of residential program. They differ from other group homes in that "these homes typically have modified programs intended to enrich their residents' later years" (Seltzer and Krauss 1987). Such programs emphasize maintaining existing abilities over trying to develop new skills, emphasize resident-initiated activities over staff-directed activities, and emphasize supporting the need for a more relaxed pace over exposing residents to new challenges (Seltzer and Krauss 1987).

Group Homes with Nurses

While attempting to maintain as typical a group home setting as possible, group homes with nurses provide more attention to the medical and health care needs of the elderly person with mental retardation. According to Seltzer and Krauss (1987), "Many have physically redesigned the program environment to accommodate the declining health of their residents"; for example, programs can eliminate problems stairways pose to the elderly by designing single-story dwellings.

When compared to other programs, group homes with nurses are characterized by the following (Seltzer and Krauss 1987):

— They are more specifically designed to serve elderly persons with mental retardation than group homes without nurses;

— They receive a higher budget per resident;

— They have a higher number of staff per resident;

— They offer a higher average number of services;

— They have a larger program size;

— They have a slightly higher percentage of elderly residents with severe and profound mental retardation than other group homes; and

— They have residents with a lower average age than that of traditional group homes.

212 | A GUIDE TO MENTAL RETARDATION

Intermediate Care Facilities for Persons with Mental Retardation (ICFs/MR)

Compared to other programs, Intermediate Care Facilities for persons with mental retardation (ICFs/MR) are characterized by the following (Seltzer and Krauss 1987):
— They have both the structure and programming to meet the needs of very challenging residents;
— They are more specifically designed, for the most part, to meet the needs of elderly persons with mental retardation than any other placement;
— They serve the highest percentage of persons with severe and profound mental retardation;
— They have the highest number of staff per resident;
— They provide the largest number of services;
— They are most likely to have a high percentage of their residents in some formal day program; and
— They are the most costly of the residential models.
In addition, "While many ICFs/MR describe themselves as capable of meeting the needs of older residents with mental retardation because of their diverse mixture of staff and service, these programs have a large number of regulation constraints" (Seltzer and Krauss 1987). The authors add: "And while the required availability of medical and nursing staff allow these programs to accept persons whose health is expected to deteriorate and for whom participation in day programming was not required, the current health of residents in these locations is no worse than in other residential models" (Seltzer and Krauss 1987).

Apartment Programs

Apartment programs are usually located in actual apartment buildings. Within this setting, staff provide less than twenty-four hours a day supervision and may either live in the apartment complex or make visits on a routine basis. The residents are usually responsible for their own housekeeping, meal preparation, and basic living skills, while the degree of assistance from staff may vary (Seltzer and Krauss 1987).
The key features of apartment programs include the following (Seltzer and Krauss 1987):

— They are more likely to use generic senior services — in other words, those services designed for the general geriatric population;

— They provide more protective supervision than formal services to residents;

— They are more likely to have residents stay home during the day; and

— These programs primarily serve residents who are more mildly retarded than do other programs.

Apartment programs, however, are less likely to be as adaptable to the changing health, emotional, and social needs of persons with mental retardation as these individuals age. Therefore, as Seltzer and Krauss (1987) have suggested, "these programs may be suitable for older persons with mental retardation who are still capable of a high level of independent functioning."

Mixed Residential Programs

Mixed residential programs are among the oldest programs. These programs often serve elderly persons with mental retardation along with nonretarded elders, where the percentage of elderly persons with mental retardation is lower in comparison. While serving the largest number of clients overall, mixed residential settings provide among the lowest average number of services, have the highest percentage of residents at home during the day with no formal program, and are the least expensive of all the models presented (Seltzer and Krauss 1987). Furthermore, these programs are the least likely to see elderly persons with mental retardation as having special needs; rather, these programs tend to be very informal both structurally and in terms of their programming (Seltzer and Krauss 1987).

The Right to Choose a Setting

According to researchers, a large percentage of aging persons with mental retardation live in supervised and restrictive residential settings, where it is believed that 30 to 40% of them do not require this level of restrictive care (Janicki and MacEachron 1984 in Edgerton 1988). Until recently, there were successful living ar-

214 | A GUIDE TO MENTAL RETARDATION

rangements among elderly persons with mental retardation in less restrictive settings.

Edgerton (1988), in a study following the lives of a sample of sixteen elderly persons with mental retardation from 1960 to the late 1980s, reveals that a majority of mildly and even moderately retarded adults can adapt successfully to community living if they are given enough time and the help of others in doing so. Given the chance to live in nonrestrictive settings, elderly persons with mental retardation would have more reciprocal relationships with nonretarded individuals; they would have a far wider range of social competencies; and they probably would have greater self-esteem as a result of their success in community living (Edgerton 1988).

If given the choice, would elderly individuals with mental retardation choose a nonrestrictive setting? Interestingly enough, according to Edgerton (1988), when older persons with mental retardation are offered opportunities to live more independently, "they often decline the offer, preferring their restrictive and routine lives to the unknown."

According to the same study by Edgerton (1988), "elderly persons with mental retardation not only fear the unknown, they typically have had little experience making choices."

"I don't think day treatment has prepared them," one worker sadly states. "We're just trying to create opportunities for making choices in our senior program.

"However, with our seniors we are dealing with people who have spent fifty years or more with no choices. What do they know from choice?

"I think there is a point for many people, regardless of age, where making choices becomes an uncomfortable imposition. A lot of older people in the normal population find having to make choices very difficult, and a lot of times you'll see the family making choices for those people — sometimes appropriate, sometimes inappropriate.

"However, there is a point, sometimes, with elderly people where their inability to make those choices has to do with their inability to accept their own limitations — for instance, limitations of aging and an inability to relate realistically to their environment.

"I don't think it is a cut-and-dried situation. If you could start with the people not going through the special education system, hopefully these individuals will have learned to make choices. And if you continue this process through their adult years, then you probably have more active seniors who can handle making choices."

Edgerton (1988), in conclusion to his study, states: "Like children, persons with mental retardation who live in restrictive settings have choices made for them. [Yet] our culture makes the right to choose for oneself a fundamental value. The right — and the necessity — to make crucial choices about one's life must be a central definition of normalization."

Finding a Specialized Day Program

Research indicates both similarities and differences in the characteristics and service needs of elderly persons with mental retardation as compared to both young adults with mental retardation and elderly nondisabled persons (Seltzer and Krauss 1987). According to Seltzer, "It is not clear from the available research whether elderly persons with mental retardation would benefit most from day programs designed for younger mentally retarded adults, from day programs for nonretarded senior citizens, or from a combination of the two."

Following is a description and comparison of day program options based upon a national survey by Seltzer and Krauss (1987).

Vocational Day Activity Programs

A vocational day activity program is a full-time program for elderly persons with mental retardation in which job-related activities are offered in the program of services (Seltzer and Krauss 1987). Such programs, in sum, are modifications of traditional day programs that aim to delay retirement for elderly persons with mental retardation.

When compared to other day program options, vocational day activity programs are one of the few programs that provide many formal services to its clients, and which provide for persons who are more severely handicapped. According to Seltzer and Krauss (1987), "Since clients in this type of program tend to be the

216 | A GUIDE TO MENTAL RETARDATION

youngest of the day program models, this service type may be the first option used when an older mentally retarded person's functional abilities begin to decline."

Day Activity Program

A day activity program is a full-time program for adults with mental retardation in which no vocational services are provided (Seltzer and Krauss 1987). Within these settings, programming tends to be self-contained, and has a relatively low level of physical and social integration with younger adults with mental retardation or nonretarded elderly persons compared to other models (Seltzer and Krauss 1987). The philosophy behind these programs, according to Seltzer and Krauss (1987), "is to provide a normalized retirement option for mentally retarded elders."

Supplemental Retirement Programs

Supplemental retirement programs, a part-time day program for elderly persons with mental retardation, clearly articulate a major objective for a retirement option. These programs tend to focus on recreational opportunities rather than vocational activities, including such activities as volunteer work, gardening, bowling, arts and crafts, cooking, sewing, and music (Seltzer and Krauss 1987).

Compared to other day treatment options, these programs have a higher rate of physical and social integration with younger adults with mental retardation and with elderly nonretarded persons, and are the most likely to use generic services for senior citizens for their own clients (Seltzer and Krauss 1987).

Leisure and Outreach Services

Programs included under this heading range from summer camps to in-home services to adult educational classes to community outings (Seltzer and Krauss 1987). These programs are typically part-time and primarily serve elderly persons with mental retardation, focused on leisure activities and/or community participation.

The benefits of leisure and outreach services are many. They offer a wide variety of creative services to elderly persons with mental retardation at a comparatively low cost, while providing a particularly important service to families through respite and in-home support (Seltzer and Krauss 1987). Compared to other options, according to Seltzer and Krauss (1987), "This model was the least integrated with the aging service network [and] was the least likely to use generic senior citizen services for their clients and to integrate elderly nonretarded clients into their programs. . . . The staff-to-client ratio is the lowest [and] they tend to include the highest functioning clients of any model."

Senior Citizen Programs

Senior citizen programs, generally, were not established for the purpose of serving elderly persons with mental retardation. However, these places do acknowledge the importance of providing services to this population (Seltzer and Krauss 1987).

According to Seltzer and Krauss (1987), at least 10% of the persons served in this program are mentally retarded, and at least half of the clients are age fifty-five or older.

Compared to other day programs, senior citizen programs have the following characteristics (Seltzer and Krauss 1987):

— They are the most unique in organizational context, program characteristics, and client characteristics;

— They have the second highest functioning clients of any model;

— The health of its clients is reportedly the most impaired; and

— They are more likely to serve persons with mental retardation who live with their families and in semi-independent apartments.

Retirement as an Option

For the general population, the proportion of an individual's life spent in retirement is on the increase. As illustrated by Seltzer and Krauss (1987), "Retirement has gained acceptability as a stage in life when the pursuit of leisure interest is sanctioned and as a time when social expectations for individual productivity decline." However, as Seltzer points out: "It is particularly striking, there-

218 | A GUIDE TO MENTAL RETARDATION

fore, that the issue of retirement for persons with mental retardation has received relatively scant attention by policymakers and service planners."

The issue of a retirement option for persons with mental retardation draws differing opinions. On one side, people may fear that "if persons with mental retardation retire, they will become passive, their skills will regress, and they will face idle, unstimulating days" (Wolfensberber 1985 in Seltzer and Krauss 1987). On the other side, there are those who believe that a retirement option should exist for persons with mental retardation just as for other older persons, feeling that as persons with mental retardation age their interest in and endurance for participation in vocational and educational day programs fade (Catapano, Levy, and Levy 1985 in Seltzer and Krauss 1987).

Retirement Due to Declining Abilities

"The choice to retire, for most people, comes from outside of themselves," one worker suggests. "In other words, they don't personally make that choice.

"It seems that most of the people who retire from the workshops do so because they either have medical disabilities that interfere with their production, or experience other problems due to aging.

"They really have a lot of anxiety in terms of not making money and not being involved in routines — all the things which helped their sense of self. They believed: 'This is the real world. I do my work — this is who I am.' Then, all of a sudden, we take that away from them.

"People in the workshops basically work as long as they are up to production. For instance, there are plenty of people in wheelchairs, and as long as they can keep up to production standards, they can still work.

"Matters are different, however, if they have incontinence problems — which are common — or if they have mobility problems, or problems with arthritis where they don't have the dexterity they once had. There are a lot of different issues. It basically comes down to lack of production; there are set requirements.

They have to meet a certain standard. If they can't meet that standard anymore, they are considered unemployable, and so have to do something else; they have to go to day treatment."

Retirement and the General Population

Many issues and trends which have evolved from studies focused on retirement for the general, nonretarded aging population have provided useful implications for the study of retirement options for elderly persons with mental retardation. First, retirement does not have to mean the abrupt end of one's employment situation; rather, it may be a process, spanning several years, in which a gradual shift in the person's work schedule and activities occurs (Seltzer and Krauss 1987).

Second, retirement does not necessarily mean the end of employment altogether; persons with mental retardation can move from full time to part time. "We're now trying to get the agency to set up a half-day program, so we will have people who do half-day day treatment and half-day workshop," one worker explains. "What is changing the focus is that day treatment can now offer paid work to day treatment service recipients: it's called Therapeutic Vocational Services. Obviously, this can't be offered all day, but it can be offered for a portion of the day so that people can be paid. In our retirement program, we will hopefully have a half day of paid work — if they choose to work.

"In addition, on this half-day schedule, people will be able to work at their own rate, get paid, and will not have to meet any kind of production standards. If they make a dollar a week, that's fine. They do the work at their own pace, as much as they want to do, and as often as they choose to do it. This is one circumstance where we are building the opportunity for choice into the program."

Third, retirement is becoming a predictable and often an eagerly anticipated time in life that offers the opportunity for more leisure and recreational activities (Seltzer and Krauss 1987). Another positive view is that the retirement of persons from the different types of day programs opens new opportunities for other persons with mental retardation to enter into those positions (Seltzer and Krauss 1987).

220 | A GUIDE TO MENTAL RETARDATION

Providing for Retirement

One important issue yet to be resolved is whether, and how, older persons with mental retardation working in sheltered workshops will be able to retire. Several advocacy groups are trying to address this problem by creating a modest retirement allowance that would replace the workshop paycheck (*The New York Times,* October 28, 1990).

Unfortunately, providing for retirement is not simple. According to an article in *The New York Times,* most retarded people depend on their Supplemental Security Income, which they would lose, under current law, if they accumulated more than $2,000 in a pension account. "Until an agreement last year between the Administration on Aging and the Administration on Developmental Disabilities," the article continues, "it was not even clear that older people with retardation were entitled to the same government services as other older Americans." The article describes how, today, many states are beginning to coordinate their services for the aging with their services for the mentally retarded (*The New York Times,* October 28, 1990).

Lack of Transition into Retirement

While efforts to provide for retirement to the elderly population of developmentally disabled adults is noteworthy, all too often many people are unprepared for the dramatic change in their routine. As one worker explains: "There is no program for transition between work and retirement; there is no preparation. I think it's tragic. A person's rights may be violated when they are taken out of the work environment and placed into, say, a day treatment location.

"For example, one individual, as a result of his declining abilities, didn't want to do anything anymore; he didn't want to work, but he also did not want to leave his work environment. Sadly, his choice was limited by the services available."

Do They Want to Retire?

While many people may assume that retirement is desirable for people with mental retardation, there actually are elderly persons with mental retardation who do not want to retire and who want to

Senior Living | 221

work. According to Kavanagh (1988), those individuals who typically say that they would like to retire actually mean that they would like to retire to more interesting jobs rather than stop working altogether.

"In many ways, this is a hard question for us to answer," one worker explains. "When people retire, they have a hard time making those kinds of choices; structuring their time, or even just making choices.

"They don't have the interests either. It's a real revelation to us to see these people in the retirement program who really don't know what to do with themselves. They lack a sense of self-direction, and they are, in general, higher functioning than the rest of the day treatment population. They haven't the foggiest idea. People have told them what to do. They've been like cogs in a machine; they've known one thing and that's all they've known" (Judy Capurso).

Yet according to another worker in the field, "that they don't know what they'd like to do with their newly found free time may not be entirely true, as I discovered one day while sitting with a group of retirees, and overheard a conversation between two gentleman concerning their dissatisfactions. Interestingly, realizing that I was listening, one gentleman became quiet.

"It wasn't long, however, after I reflected some of the comments back to them that I had overheard, that both gentleman continued their conversation to include me: 'We never get paid,' one man continued. 'We never get to carry our own money. I'd like to have my own money so I can buy what I want.' Being the more vocal of the two, he continued to express his unhappiness about the program: 'We don't do anything here. We don't do anything at our house. We just sit there, and they play the television. I would just like to go out bowling sometime, or go to the park. But we don't do these things.' "

Creating Meaning in Their Lives

One thing that is important is that these people need to perceive that there is something positive about choosing a certain activity. As one worker tells: "A lot of times, I think we railroad people into doing certain things because we think it would be a good experience. They, however, don't really get anything out of the

222 | A GUIDE TO MENTAL RETARDATION

experience. They don't know what they are supposed to feel; we don't exactly know how to tailor the experience so that they get something meaningful out of it. And so, making choices becomes our preoccupation; not something that gives them fulfillment.

"That's why people might be more excited about having choices if they actually got something out of the activity. They have to perceive something. For instance, there are certain people in our program who love to sing, and they would choose that if they were offered something to do. During our leisure time, there are a few women who love to sew — they are obsessed with sewing, and they would sew everyday. You can see that they're really enjoying it. This is not an artificial *filler* for the day. They're not just doing it because we've asked them to do it. Unfortunately, they are used to being told what to do; they're used to being compliant."

Counseling Issues

On Death and Dying

As I grow older, the reality that my parents have already moved into their senior years has become alarmingly real. While at one time I may have believed that they would be alive forever, I now am discovering that my time with them is becoming shorter and shorter, and as a result, more precious to me.

My attachment with the elderly persons I work with, while not as intense as the relationship with my parents, is nonetheless just as valid. And the longer I work with them, and the more fragile their lives become, the more sensitive I am to my own feelings about their death, either suddenly or after a period of hospitalization.

I then wonder: How does this affect people who are retarded? How do they interpret death? What do they need to help them through mourning the death of a parent, sibling, friend, peer?

"I don't think their needs are any different than somebody who doesn't have a disability," one worker feels. "These are questions for which there are no satisfying answers. You're not going to get this person back. But they can have the chance to explore those feelings, to be allowed to have those feelings, to have somebody talk with them about those feelings. At one of our senior residences, this is a constant issue because people are dying."

Only just recently, a very sweet old woman, Helen, had passed away. While this is not the first person at my agency who has died, she is one of the first that I can recall where the agency clearly made an effort to provide some form of closure for the remaining family members, staff, and especially her peers through a memorial service. It was a clear way of saying goodbye and paying our last respects.

"We had a gentleman from a local funeral home come into our senior facility to make a presentation to the staff and residents," one worker describes. "He got the group involved in exploring their feelings."

"I worked in a workshop where someone had died," another worker tells, noticing how much more humanistic facilities have become. "We closed shop, and everyone went to the funeral. One of the staff said to me, 'This is a lot different than when I first came here about eight years ago. A person had died, and the staff told the clients that this person had moved away and wasn't coming back anymore.' "

Some individuals have no family contact, and so are unaware when a parent or sibling has died. For others, by decision of a treatment team, the facts may be kept from them due to fears of negative reactions and behaviors.

Abandonment

"You can't work in the field without seeing all of these examples of people abandoned by their family," one worker explains. "It's not just the older people who are institutionalized when that was the thing to do; it still happens to some extent.

"I was working with one young gentleman, and it was shocking. He is so charming; he has such a winning personality. I personally doubt his diagnosis of mental retardation — instead, I think he was environmentally deprived. And yet, he was abandoned by his family. His family lives fairly close, and they visit him once a year. He's in heaven when they come to take him for lunch for an hour once a year.

"Even working with people who are very low functioning, there is this inarticulate, emotional cry, even forty years after being

224 | A GUIDE TO MENTAL RETARDATION

abandoned by the family; they still have a desperate need at holidays when everyone else has family contact — at holidays, they are full of despair."

"One woman lived with her family up to a certain point in her life," another worker continues, "and every holiday she experiences this incredible anxiety. She talks over and over about some member of her family, 'Gee, I'd really like to go home for Christmas. Well, I know she's really busy. Are they going to get in touch with me? Am I going to get to go home? Should I expect a visit? Should I expect a card?' It really breaks my heart to watch her go through this."

Regardless of how long it's been since these people last saw that familiar face from years ago, the memories still lie waiting. "I don't think you can replace that family involvement and that primary tie," one worker expresses. "The emotional impact of that primary tie is so incredibly important, no matter what level of developmental disability. The loss of the primary tie becomes a central feature in their lives — and it's so traumatic.

"Even with our seniors — we have people who may seem to have grown beyond expressing this need to see their families, but emotionally this is still extremely important. Even if it's just a niece or nephew, however distant the relationship, that is their family. No matter whether they are seventy or thirty-five, that is still the primary focus of their emotional life."

Effect on Institutionalized Person

For individuals who may never have had any significant contact with family, especially those whose lives have been spent in institutions, the feelings of abandonment, while sometimes not as apparent, can be just as intense. As one worker tells: "There are some people who were abandoned so long ago — from the age of four or five they've been in an institution. They didn't have any family contact; that has not been a feature of their life at all. You could say that they have a loss of affect or something; they just don't get emotional about human interaction to the same extent.

"Some may develop surrogate bonds though. If they form close ties with staff people, or if they have sustained emotional relationships with a person with whom they identify in that same way — someone who protects you, someone who loves you unconditionally; all the things we identify as parental.

"For example, one woman, Regina, mothers some of her peers. Even today, she mothers one woman who is thirty-five-years-old, but Regina perceives her role with this younger woman as mothering. Regina says that 'she's my baby.' They've known each other for many years at the institutions."

Regulations: How They Can Destroy Relationships

Regulations, while a means to ensure that a system runs smoothly and consistently, may also disrupt some basic human needs all people have to maintain a sense of mental health. As one worker recalls: "I worked with a woman in an institution who, years ago, had been in a group of other women. They had lived together for years and they were all very high functioning. At one point, their hall was broken up and they were separated. Several of them died within six months.

"Afterwards, the state auditors were after us to place this woman in the community. She was extremely resistant; she didn't want to go. She was very high functioning and able to make her own decisions. Her family even begged us, 'Don't take her away. She's over seventy. This has been her life since she was about twenty-two. It will kill her.' I demanded that the auditor talk to the woman, but because of some regulation, the response was 'No, it says here on forms x, y, and z that you have to refer her to the community.'

"The state sets itself up to constantly intervene on behalf of a person for a less restrictive environment. But if a person is already functioning very well in a situation and all of a sudden there is an opening out in the community, do you arbitrarily remove that person from a very good situation to meet an artificial standard? Is there any humanity involved here? Instead, we should move somebody to a less restrictive environment for the right reasons, not for a completely arbitrary reason."

"Another example," another worker shares. "A while ago, an individual was to be moved out of her residential placement into a family care home — but before the move, so much emotion was expressed by the residential staff. 'Yes, she's moving to a less restrictive environment. Sure, she'll get her own wheelchair ramp

226 | A GUIDE TO MENTAL RETARDATION

and modified bathroom. But think of the friendships she'll be leaving behind. She'll be losing the things that are most meaningful to her.' There was the concern of her being isolated in this family setting.

"It was a very hot issue. And the issues that were brought up were not really resolved. This was a case where she may not be aware of her rights; she may not necessarily be aware of what she's giving up.

"She now lives in a situation where she gets a tremendous amount of one-to-one attention and intervention, and receives a lot of things because she is the focus of the family care provider's responsibility and affections. But she no longer hangs out with people of her own ethnicity. She no longer hangs out with her peers."

Medical Issues

As a result of their increased life span, many persons with developmental disabilities are now facing problems related to old age.

Receiving Treatment

The paucity of available practitioners who are willing to work with the developmentally disabled population is surprising. Kavanagh (1988) describes the following: "In general, those persons with mental retardation who live into old age are quite healthy and sturdy. Their problems of medical care are for the most part problems of access, for they tend to be not much valued as individuals by generic service providers. Nor do community physicians feel that they are adequately rewarded by Medicaid for provision of services to this population."

With deinstitutionalization, one worker believes that the people who moved away from the institutions, ironically, lost willing practitioners who were located near the institution: "The one positive thing about residence in an institution was the level of medical care. The medical staff were all experts in the field of developmental disabilities. There was a psychiatrist on staff, someone who could deal very well with the unique problems that exist for this population.

"However, when I was working in community services and we were taking our people to the hospital, we couldn't get services. We would take our people to the emergency room, and doctors would say, 'This person doesn't have a mental illness; he has mental retardation.'

"One doctor who had fairly recently come to work with the mentally retarded population said, 'I had no idea. My colleagues have no idea what this population is like. They had never heard of dual diagnosis.' "

While the unfamiliarity with the developmentally disabled population may be one factor making it difficult to find a willing practitioner, payment is another. As one worker describes: "There were times when we had this massive search for a dentist. There's a whole country from which to choose, yet we couldn't find one dentist who would take Medicaid patients. Or else they did it at one time, but they don't anymore because the Medicaid system is so problematic itself that professional people don't want to deal with it.

"For example, we found a good dentist at one time, but eventually he said, 'I can't take any more of your clients.' In addition, he later called us and asked, 'Could you please write to Medicaid for me so that I might get paid for my services?' "

"This is a classic complaint of Medicaid: Either you don't get paid adequately, you don't get paid on time, or you'll do a service and Medicaid will deny its having been done," another worker elaborates.

"For example, if a certain set of x-rays reveal the need for emergency dental work, you'll go ahead with the procedure. Obviously, if you're compassionate enough, you'll go ahead with the operation; you won't let someone sit around with an abscess for three weeks while you get Medicaid approval. Unfortunately, the attitude we get in return it, 'You should have just pulled the tooth. You shouldn't have done a root canal. Don't try to save the tooth.' Medicaid would rather pull the tooth out because it cost too much to fix, or else they won't approve the surgery. However, it doesn't seem like they are concerned that this individual may wish to save their tooth.

228 | A GUIDE TO MENTAL RETARDATION

"As a result, the dental hygiene of most of our adult and senior individuals is disastrous. Why hadn't someone intervened years ago? Most of our adults could look a lot better than they do if only they had a little oral surgery."

Dementia and Mental Retardation

Individuals with mental retardation develop dementia from the same causes as the general population (Barcikowska, Silverman, Zigman, Kozlowski, Kujawa, Rudelli, and Wisniewski 1989). "As medical science prolongs the life span of persons with mental retardation," one author notes, "diagnosing and treating dementia in persons with mental retardation has become an increasingly important clinical area" (Hurley and Sovner 1986).

Diagnosis

According to Barcikowska et al. (1989), dementia is extremely difficult to diagnose in persons with mental retardation. Often, dementia is misdiagnosed as a psychological or behavioral problem, and the individual is often referred to a psychologist or behavioral specialist; as a result, the underlying medical pathology is missed.

With this in mind, sensitivity to the causes for declining behavior should occur before assuming Alzheimer's disease or dementia, since the signs of such behavior may result in transfers out of a group home and workshop into a nursing home. As Kavanagh (1988) has suggested, other causes for decreased behavior should be considered. The individual with mental retardation may be grieving due to the death or absence of a parent or sibling, staff member or friend. They also may be mourning changes which may have occurred in their residence or workshop. Furthermore, physical changes, such as a decrease in exercise tolerance, arthritic pain, or a decrease in sensory acuity may create behavioral changes resembling those seen in Alzheimer's disease.

To ensure that the diagnosis of dementia is not missed, Hurley and Sovner (1986) recommend that any mentally retarded individual referred for a behavioral-psychological problem also be tested for intelligence. If any loss of cognitive functioning is detected, a referral to a neurologist and/or neuropsychologist for further evaluation should be considered (Hurley and Sovner 1986).

Down Syndrome and Alzheimer's Disease

There is an extremely high incidence of Alzheimer's disease among persons with Down syndrome (Wisniewski, Wisniewski, and Wen 1985 in Zigman, Schuff, Lubin, and Silverman 1987). While the percentage of Alzheimer's disease among persons with mental retardation is similar to that of the general population (Barcikowska et al. 1989), research indicates that Alzheimer's disease strikes people with Down syndrome during their thirties and forties (Hurley and Sovner 1986), while other researchers suggest a later onset, between age forty and fifty (Zigman et al. 1987).

This higher incidence may be related to the fact that the physical and functional capacities of people with Down syndrome, regardless of developmental level, appear to decline with age at an accelerated rate (Zigman et al. 1987). Evidence of premature aging includes the increased prevalence of diseases related to old age, including certain types of cancer, degenerative vascular disease, diabetes mellitus, cataracts, and gray hair (Balacz 1985 in Hurley et al. 1986).

The life expectancy of persons with Down syndrome who lacked mobility or eating skills has been found to be poor as compared to individuals who have Down syndrome but did not have these programs regardless of the presence of heart disease.

Appendix A

The Medicaid Waiver

The Medicaid Waiver is a funding mechanism designed to provide a variety of services for individuals with mental retardation. Rather then offering a package of services that might not mesh with the individual's needs, the Medicaid Waiver allows the case manager and the client to design a unique program.

The following is taken from an interview with Peter Pierri, Executive Director of Ulster ARC in Kingston, New York.

Q: What is the general idea for the Medicaid Waiver?

The Medicaid Waiver, in a general sense, is a new source of funding which will help us provide services for people that cannot get these services in the current system.

More importantly, for workers in the field who are deeply involved in the current system, the Medicaid Waiver is a new way of thinking. It is important to realize that this is not just a new program, or a new way of providing services. It is a whole new way of thinking for service providers. To some degree, we are going to have to forget how we have been doing things; we have to start thinking in a new way.

Q: How was the Waiver approved in New York State?

232 | A GUIDE TO MENTAL RETARDATION

The state of New York applied for and received approval from the federal government for a waiver from certain Medicaid restrictions.

Up to that point in New York State, the way Medicaid funding could be used for people with disabilities was primarily in two ways. Medicaid pays for services in the day treatment program, and Medicaid also pays for services in Intermediate Care Facilities (ICFs). Other than this, we could not use Medicaid monies for services for people with disabilities — outside of a regular physician, medical treatment, and so on.

The application that the state of New York submitted to the federal government was expected to waive some of those federal restrictions. We told the state that we wanted to be able to use Medicaid monies in a variety of different ways and a variety of different locations; not just in those specific programs. And we are convinced that we can serve more people for the same amount of money. We received approval in October 1991.

One reason the state is interested in getting this program off the ground is the financial benefit. The state is going to be able to use Medicaid services for people who are currently receiving services differently.

Medicaid is a program where 50% of all Medicaid money comes from the federal government, and 50% comes from the state government. So if New York State has a way of getting more federal money to provide services rather than state money, this would help New York State's budget. At the same time, the state will be able to provide services to more people than they could have before. It's sort of a win-win situation.

The state of New York is not really so revolutionary. Actually, this state is very much behind the times. There are at least forty other states which already have received approval from the federal government, and have been operating programs in this way for a very long time.

Q: Who is eligible for the Medicaid Waiver?

Medicaid Waiver programs throughout the country are granted a certain number of slots — I think it's from 1,100 to 1,700 slots for New York State this year. That means the federal government will allot New York State monies to provide Medicaid Waivered services to up to 1,700 people during the coming year.

The person with a disability is able to receive services under the Medicaid Waiver regardless of the program in which they are enrolled or where they may be living. However, the individual needs to be Medicaid eligible, and they have to have a disability which is severe enough to make them eligible for an Intermediate Care Facility (ICF).

The actual regulations specifying eligibility requirements for someone to be in an ICF are very, very broad, and very, very loose. The way we at ARC happened to have structured our programs, most of the people who live in our ICFs are people with severe disabilities. The fact of the matter is that about 80% of the people who live in our Community Residence program (CR) also meet the typical ICF requirements; it's just that we have chosen to place these people in less restrictive homes than ones which they are actually eligible for.

Basically, the person has to have a diagnosis of a developmental disability — which is mental retardation, cerebral palsy, epilepsy, neurological impairment, or autism — and also have a significant disability in the area of self-care — hygiene, communication, and so on.

When people hear that the individual has to be eligible for an ICF in order to qualify for a Waiver slot, some people automatically have a picture in their minds that the person may not qualify because he or she is not handicapped enough. But in all likelihood, many of the people in ARC programs would qualify for ICF-level of care, and therefore would qualify for a Waiver slot.

Some of the people who live in our Supportive Apartments may *not* qualify because they may have certain life skills which would make them ineligible. Some people receiving Supportive Employment from ARC may, or may not, be eligible; it depends upon their total level of disability in specific areas.

Most of our clients who receive services at ARC are already Medicaid eligible. In order to qualify for Medicaid, two criteria need to be met. One is the level of disability, which is determined as a long-term disability which makes that individual person dependent on others. The other aspect of Medicaid eligibility is financial. Most of the people who attend ARC programs do not have assets or money which would make them Medicaid ineligible. However, the group that is often found Medicaid ineligible is children; in New York State the parental income — not the child's income — is used to determine their eligibility for Medicaid.

234 | A GUIDE TO MENTAL RETARDATION

Under the Medicaid Waiver, that restriction is waived. It means that a child who had a disability who would otherwise be eligible for Medicaid, but cannot get Medicaid due to the parent's income, can receive services under the Medicaid Waiver *regardless of his parent's income.*

For the first time, disabled children who are living at home will be eligible for assistance regardless of the parent's financial status.

Q: What are the services available under the Medicaid Waiver?

There are eight services available under the Medicaid Waiver: Case Management, Residential Habilitation, Day Habilitation Services, Environmental Modification, Respite, Supportive Employment, Prevocational Employment, and Adaptive Technology. These are the only services that the Medicaid Waiver program pays for.

Case Management

Out of the eight service areas, Case Management is the only service that is absolutely required. If the person does not receive Case Management services, they cannot get any other services under the Waiver.

Case Management under the Waiver is very different from what we generally consider as case management. The agency who provides case management services to the consumer is the most important service provider in the program. They are responsible for helping to put together the Individual's Service Plan (ISP). The whole concept of the Medicaid Waiver is to establish individualized services for people.

The case manager works with the consumer in determining what services the consumer needs. From there, a service plan is made with that consumer. The Medicaid Waiver is based upon the individuals making choices for themselves and initiating the request for services. The case manager, in essence, works *for the consumer,* and is the procurer of services for the consumer.

Residential Habilitation

The first kind of service that the case manager can procure for the consumer is Residential Habilitation. Basically, this entails services

The Medicaid Waiver | 235

that take place in the person's living environment; they involve training which will aid the individual in his or her independence and growth. This can be in the areas of hygiene, grooming, socialization, recreation — general habilitative services similar to what ARC provides now within its programs.

In order to receive Residential Habilitaive services, a consumer can live almost anywhere *except* an ICF. The case manager can procure Residential Habilitative services in an apartment setting, in a family care home, in the person's own home, in a home where there happen to be four other people with disabilities, or in a home where there are two people with disabilities and two people without disabilities.

The services are not tied to a building; instead they are geared toward the individual. Under the Waiver, the services are very prescriptive and very individualized.

Conceptually, under the Waiver, as the person becomes more independent, he or she doesn't have to leave the house. Today we have people moving from an ICF to a CR to a supervised apartment to a supportive apartment — if they can get this far. In the past we've told our clients: you've done so well, and so now you are going to have to move; you are going to leave your friends, your neighborhood, your community. Of course this is counterproductive. However, it has happened in the past because services and programs have been seen as one entity.

It will all be reversed under the Medicaid Waiver. It's all changing. The services are not tied to a person's living environment; they are tied to the person's needs. So the person can stay where he or she wants, and the services can be adapted as that person's needs change.

Day Habilitation Services

There are also Day Habilitation Services which are available for the consumer. Day Habilitation is essentially the same as Residential Habilitation, only it occurs in a location other than one's living environment. Day Habilitation programs teach people independent living skills, recreation and socialization skills, structured activities — things that are not necessarily addressed in the home. For example, under Day Habilitation services, a case manager could help arrange for the consumer to volunteer at a nursing

236 | A GUIDE TO MENTAL RETARDATION

home for three hours a day. Or the case manager could arrange for someone to work with the consumer on their food shopping on Thursday evenings; or teaching the consumer how to take a city bus to get to the movies by themselves, or to look in the newspaper to find out what recreation is available in town. And and all of these kinds of things can be considered day habilitation.

Environmental Modification

Under the Waiver, one of the things that a case manager can do for the consumer is arrange for actual physical changes to the home in which that person lives. If the person's disability is such that changes to the home would make them more independent, funding can be requested.

For example, if a person's physical condition has deteriorated to where they are in a wheelchair, and they have four steps that go up to their house — under the Waiver, the case manager can request funding for environmental services to build a ramp up to the house.

Respite

Respite services allow families to have time for vacations or other planned activities. Currently, through Family Support Services, we have a good respite program. The Waiver, however, will be able to enhance those services by increasing the opportunity to pay for these services.

Supportive Employment and Prevocational Training

Because of the federal government requirements under Medicaid, Supportive Employment and Prevocational Training are available under the Waiver *only if the consumer has at some point lived in an ICF.* This is not to say that the case manager can't arrange for supportive employment for someone who was never in an ICF. It just means that the Medicaid Waiver program will not be paying for that service.

Prevocational training, which is very similar to the programming in day treatment, can be procured by the case manager without the person being in a day treatment program.

The Medicaid Waiver | 237

Adaptive Technology

Adaptive technology can include personal emergency response systems, various types of communicators and speech amplifiers, standing boards and frames, motorized wheelchairs, and guide dogs. Anything adaptive that aids the individual's independence and growth can be a service that will be paid for by the Medicaid Waiver. (Note: For a catalogue on adaptive equipment, call 1-800-221-6827.)

Q: How does the Medicaid Waiver affect other services?

The Medicaid Waiver is a New York State Medicaid program which does not replace or supplant — it is not allowed to replace or supplant — any services that are listed under the State Use Plan. The State Use Plan under Medicaid is anything you can buy with your Medicaid card.

Q: Will the Waiver assist in transportation to services?

Transportation is not a Medicaid Waiver service. However, transportation to a Medicaid funded service is reimbursable in the state of New York by Medicaid.

As an agency, we are a Medicaid transportation vendor; we have a Medicaid number strictly for our transportation services. We can get reimbursed by Medicaid for transporting our people to day treatment. But if we transport our people to Pilot Industries, we do not get reimbursed by Medicaid because it is not a Medicaid-funded service to which they are going.

Individual Service Plan

The case manager writes the Individual Service Plan *with* the consumer — not *for* the consumer — and they determine together what kind of service the person wants and needs. That plan is them submitted through the agency to the Developmental Disability Service Office (DDSO) for approval.

The Medicaid Waiver can be complicated, because the services are not predetermined. Clinical teams and treatment teams have no

238 | A GUIDE TO MENTAL RETARDATION

application in the Medicaid Waiver program. There is no predetermined clinical team because the individual may not need one. The Medicaid Waiver is a system of delivering services; not a system of monitoring goals.

Clinical Services

There are two reasons it makes good sense for our ARC program to develop our own clinical department. The state has set up programs to allow us to get some Medicaid reimbursements for clinical services; therefore, we are going to have our own licensed Medicaid clinic. But it also fits in, conceptually, with the Medicaid Waiver: that services are separate from the way individuals live or what individuals do during the day.

So if we now have one clinic for the agency, a case manager will be able under the Waiver program to get speech therapy for the consumer. They don't have to be in a day treatment program in order to get speech therapy; they don't have to live in an ICF for psychological services; they can get services needed separate from the program in which they are involved. We are no longer talking about *programs*; we are talking about *services*.

Quality Assurance

The quality assurance certification is being developed, and it is going to be very different from anything else we've seen before. The quality assurance process will involve review with the case manager of the services the consumer wanted, and then follow-up to verify that those services were provided.

Part of the process will include the agencies' own internal quality assurance program. Agencies will need to prove to the state that they are doing their own quality assurance checks — and that is part of the certification. There will also be a consumer satisfaction survey — a major part of the quality assurance review of the Waiver program is going to be asking the consumers if the service provider is doing a good job for them.

Guiding Principles of the Waiver Program

The guiding principles of the Waiver program include: Individual choice, Integration, Independence, and Productivity.

The Medicaid Waiver | 239

Individual Choice

The whole shift in thinking is that everything starts with the consumer's choice. The concept of choice is emphasized so much that the consumer will even have the choice of who their case manager will be, because the case manager works for them. They will have the choice of what agency they go to. Some of these services may be met through ARC; some of them may not. It may be more appropriate for them to receive respite from the Mental Health Association. The entire process begins with the consumer's first choice.

At an in-service, one parent described her feelings about this new way of thinking. She said, "For the first time in my life, I didn't get a report which told me what my daughter could not do. I didn't get a report that listed her deficits. No one told me what was wrong with my daughter. Instead, the people started with what my daughter likes to do, what she can do, what she wants to do, and how they could help her to do these things better and more often."

There will eventually be a process — in some form — of representation for consumers who don't have their families or anyone else to advocate for them. But the Medicaid Waiver is not based upon giving informed consent. It is based upon a principle — not a legalistic regulation — but the principle that everything done under the Waiver should, if at all possible, originate from the consumer's choice. It does *not* originate from a treatment team's assessment of the person's strengths and needs. This is the major difference.

Integration

When the case manager procures any service for the consumer — whether paid for by the Medicaid Waiver program or through some other program — the case manager should ascertain that the service was what the consumer wanted, and ask the important question: *Is this going to aid the person's integration into a normal living environment in the community?*

For example, if given a choice of riding in an ARC van or a public bus, the case manager should first be thinking in terms of the public bus. Maybe it cannot be organized, and that's okay. If they are trying to arrange to do volunteer, the case manager

240 | A GUIDE TO MENTAL RETARDATION

should try to get them volunteer work where you or I would do volunteer work. If we are going to arrange for them to attend a dance, let's try to get them involved in a town dance, instead of a dance held in the ARC cafeteria.

Independence

All the services that are procured for the consumer under the Medicaid Waiver program should promote the consumer's independence.

Productivity

The Medicaid Waiver guidelines are concerned with work productivity and personal productivity: how these services aid the individuals feeling more productive in their lives. We tend to think of productivity in terms of x number of widgets they can make in a given day, which *is* part of productivity, in terms of one's work environment. But our world does not end at four o'clock. We are all productive in our lives, whether we are at work or occupied in other facets of our lives.

Regulations

In general, the system is loosening all of the regulations even in terms of the kinds of homes we are going to be allowed to open. The regulations for opening up a home with fewer than eight beds will now be no more rigid than regulations for operating a family care home. It will be substantially easier to open smaller homes with very, very few regulations in a shorter amount of time.

Protective Oversight

It will be hard for us to really allow people to make choices. It will be hard, first of all, to train and teach our people how to *make* choices. We also have a responsibility to guide them through their choices: we call this Protective Oversight. We have to be careful that we don't allow people to place themselves in situations of danger or of obvious harm. They are still people who have disabilities, and we as professionals have the responsibility for teaching them to make choices that will not harm them.

Appendix B

Excerpts from Public Law

The Education of the Handicapped Act (EHA) is also referred to as the EAHCA (Education for All Handicapped Children Act). It was changed by act of Congress to the Individuals with Disabilities Education Act (IDEA) as of October 30, 1990.

The Education of the Handicapped Act (20 USCS §§ 1401 et seq.) provides federal money to assist state and local agencies in educating handicapped children. To qualify for federal assistance, a state must demonstrate, through a detailed plan submitted for federal approval, that it has a policy in effect that assures all handicapped children the right to a free appropriate public education, which policy must be tailored to the unique needs of the handicapped child by the means of an individualized educational program (IEP). The IEP must be prepared and reviewed at least annually by school officials with participation by the child's parents or guardian. The Act also requires that a participating state provide specified administrative procedures by which the child's parents or guardian may challenge any change in the evaluation and education of the child. Any party aggrieved by the state administrative decisions is authorized to bring a civil action in either a state court or a Federal District Court.

244 | A GUIDE TO MENTAL RETARDATION

Individuals with Disabilities Education Act (IDEA)

20 USCS § 1400. Congressional statements and declarations

Findings
(1) there are more than eight million children with disabilities in the United States today;
(2) the special educational needs of such children are not being fully met;
(3) more than half of the children with disabilities in the United States do not receive appropriate educational services which would enable them to have full equality of opportunity;
(4) one million of the children with disabilities in the United States are excluded entirely from the public school system and will not go through the educational process with their peers;
(5) there are many children with disabilities throughout the United States participating in regular school programs whose disabilities prevent them from having a successful educational experience because their disabilities are undetected;
(6) because of the lack of adequate services within the public school system, families are often forced to find services outside the public school system, often at great distance from their residence and at their own expense;
(7) developments in the training of teachers and in diagnostic and instructional procedures and methods have advanced to the point that, given appropriate funding, State and local educational agencies can and will provide effective special education and related services to meet the needs of children with disabilities;
(8) State and local educational agencies have a responsibility to provide education for all children with disabilities, but present financial resources are inadequate to meet the special educational needs of children with disabilities; and
(9) it is in the national interest that the Federal Government assist State and local efforts to provide programs to meet the educational needs of children with disabilities in order to assure equal protection of the law.

Purpose. It is the purpose of this Act to assure that all children with disabilities have available to them, within the time periods specified in section 612(2)(B) [20 USCS § 1412 (2)(B)], a free appropriate public education which emphasizes special education

Excerpts from Public Law | 245

and related services designed to meet their unique needs, to assure that the rights of children with disabilities and their parents or guardians are protected, to assist States and localities to provide for the education of all children with disabilities, and to assess and assure the effectiveness of efforts to educate children with disabilities.

§ *11:25. General standard of ages 3–21.* In order for a state to be eligible for assistance in any fiscal year, a state generally must make available a free appropriate public education, for all children with disabilities between the ages of 3 and 21 within the state.

§ *11:27. Basic definition.* The term free appropriate public education means special education and related services that (1) have been provided at public expense, under public supervision and direction, and without charge; (2) meet the standards of the state educational agency; (3) include an appropriate preschool, elementary, or secondary school in the state involved; and (4) are provided in conformity with the requirement for an individualized education program (IEP).

§ *11:30. Required level of benefit to, and progress by, child.* There is no requirement that the specialized educational services provided by a state under the IDEA to a child with a disability must be sufficient to maximize the child's potential commensurate with the opportunity provided other children. Instead, a state satisfies the requirement to provide a free appropriate public education by providing personalized instruction with sufficient support services to permit the child to benefit educationally from the instruction. The instruction and services must be provided at public expense, must meet the state's educational standards, must approximate the grade levels used in the state's regular education, and must comport with the child's individualized education program (IEP). In addition, the IEP, and therefore the personalized instruction, should be formulated in accordance with the IDEA's requirements, and, if the child is being educated in the regular classrooms of the public education system, should be reasonably calculated to enable the child to achieve passing marks and advance from grade to grade. Although not every child who is advancing from grade to grade in a regular public school system is automatically receiving a free appropriate public education, the

246 | A GUIDE TO MENTAL RETARDATION

child's academic progress, when considered with the special services and consideration afforded by the school's administrators, may be dispositive in a particular case.

In general, an appropriate education is one which allows the child to make educational progress. The IDEA demands more than minimal or trivial progress, and the amount of appropriate advancement varies depending on the individual student. However, a child with disabilities who is not receiving passing marks and is not reasonably advancing from grade to grade is not necessarily being deprived of a free appropriate public education, as some children may never be able to do so, despite efforts by the state.

§ 11:31. *Basic definition of special education.* The term special education means specially designed education, at no cost to parents or guardians, to meet the needs of a child with a disability, including (1) instruction conducted in the classroom, in the home, in hospitals and institutions, and in other settings; and (2) instruction in physical education. The term special education includes speech pathology, or any other related service, if the service (1) consists of specially designed instruction, at no cost to the parents, to meet the unique needs of a child with a disability; and (2) is considered special education rather than a related service under state standards. In addition, the term includes vocational education.

The concept of special education is broad, encompassing not only traditional cognitive skills, but also basic functional skills. For children with severe disabilities, education may include the most elemental of life skills.

§ 11:33. *Vocational education.* Special education includes vocational education if it consists of specially designed instruction, at no cost to the parents, to meet the unique needs of a child with a disability. Thus, vocational education programs must be specially designed if necessary to enable a student with a disability to benefit fully from those programs. In addition, each public agency will take steps to insure that its children with disabilities have available to them the variety of vocational educational programs available to children without disabilities in the area served by the agency.

For purposes of providing special education, vocational education means organized educational programs which are directly related to the preparation of individuals for paid or unpaid employment, or for additional preparation for a career requiring other than a baccalaureate or advanced degree.

§ *11:51. Basic requirement.* In order to be eligible for general assistance under Part B of the IDEA in any fiscal year, each state must demonstrate to the Secretary of Education that the state has procedures to assure that, to the maximum extent appropriate, children with disabilities, including children in public or private institutions or other care facilities, are educated with children who are not disabled, and that special classes, separate schooling, or other removal of children with disabilities from the regular educational environment occurs only when the nature of the severity is such that education in regular classes with the use of supplementary aids and services cannot be achieved satisfactorily. This requirement is known as the least restrictive environment or mainstreaming requirement.

§ *11:63. Definition and purpose of IEP.* An individualized education program (IEP) means a written statement for each child with a disability developed in any meeting by a representative of the local educational agency or an intermediate educational unit who is qualified to provide or supervise the provision of specially designed instruction to meet the unique needs of children with disabilities, the teacher, the parents or guardian of the child, and, whenever appropriate, the child, which statement will include specified contents.

For purposes of the IDEA, the individualized education program (IEP) has been called the statute's modus operandi, the primary vehicle for implementing congressional goals, and the centerpiece of the statute's educational delivery system. The free appropriate public education required by the statute is tailored to the unique needs of a child with a disability by means of the IEP. The purposes and functions of the IEP requirement are (1) to serve as a communication and joint decision vehicle for parents and school personnel; (2) to provide an opportunity for resolving any differences between the parents and the agency; (3) to set forth in writing a commitment of necessary resources; (4) to provide a management tool; (5) to provide a compliance/monitoring document; and (6) to serve as a device in evaluating a child's progress.

248 | A GUIDE TO MENTAL RETARDATION

§ 11:66. When IEP must be in effect. At the beginning of each school year, each public agency must have in effect an individualized education program (IEP) for every child who is receiving special education from that agency. An IEP must be in effect before special education and related services are provided to a child. The term "be in effect" means that the IEP has been developed properly, is regarded by both the parent and agency as appropriate in terms of the child's needs, specified goals and objectives, and services to be provided, and will be implemented as written.

In general, IEP objectives must be written before placement. For a child with a disability receiving special education for the first time, an IEP must be developed before placement, although an eligible child may temporarily be placed in a program as part of the evaluation process before the IEP is finalized.

§ 11:140. What are early intervention services. Early intervention services are services which (1) are provided under public supervision; (2) are provided at no cost, except where federal or state law provides for a system of payments by families, including a schedule of sliding fees; (3) are designed to meet the developmental needs of an infant or toddler with a disability in one or more of the areas of physical development, cognitive development, communication development, social or emotional development, or adaptive development; (4) meet the standards of the state, including the requirements of Part H of the IDEA; (5) are among a number of specified types; (6) are provided by qualified personnel; (7) to the maximum extent appropriate, are provided in natural environments including the home, and community settings in which children without disabilities participate; and (8) are provided in conformity with a properly adopted individualized family services plan.

The types of services to be provided include (1) family training, counseling, and home visits; (2) special instruction; (3) speech pathology and audiology; (4) occupational therapy; (5) physical therapy; (6) psychological services; (7) case management services, also referred to as service coordination services; (8) medical services for diagnostic or evaluation purposes only; (9) early identification, screening, and assessment services (10) health services necessary to enable the infant or toddler to benefit from other early intervention services; (11) social work services; (12)

vision services; (13) assistive technology devices and assistive technology services; and (14) transportation and related costs that are necessary to enable an infant or toddler and the infant's or toddler's family to receive early intervention services.

§ 11:141. Assessments; individualized family service plans. Each infant or toddler with a disability and the infant's or toddler's family must receive (1) a multidisciplinary assessment of unique strengths and needs of the infant or toddler and the identification of services appropriate to meet those needs; (2) a family-directed assessment of the resources, priorities, and concerns of the family, and the identification of the supports and services necessary to enhance the family's capacity to meet the developmental needs of their infant or toddler; and (3) a written individualized family service plan, developed by a multidisciplinary team, including the parents or guardians, within a reasonable time after the assessment.

Recommended Resources

Chapter 2

There are now so many books and articles on early intervention with infants and young children with mental retardation it is difficult to maintain a current reference list. Parents may find the following books helpful:

Robin Simons, *After the Tears.* San Diego: Harcourt, Brace Jovanovich, 1987.

Ann P. Turnbull and H. Rutherford Turnbull, III, *Families, Professionals, and Exceptionality: A Special Partnership.* Columbus, OH: Merrill, 1990. This is a large and detailed book designed for professionals, but it also has many practical suggestions which parents may find helpful.

Cliff Cunningham and Patricia Sloper, *Helping Your Exceptional Baby.* New York: Pantheon Books, 1980. This book is somewhat dated now, and because it was originally published in the United Kingdom the authors naturally use British terminology, some of which may be unfamiliar to American readers. In spite of this, the book is full of practical information on the development of infants and young children, as well as activities that parents can do at home to stimulate an infant or toddler with a handicap. The activities in this book will be especially helpful in conjunction with a good early intervention program.

Bruce Baker and Alan Brightman, *Steps to Independence* (1989). A very practical guide for parents to use at home, teaching basic self-care and other important skills. Much of the book is more relevant for school-age children, but some of the skills involved in "paying attention" and "following direction" discussed in the book are relevant for toddlers.

252 | THE GUIDE TO MENTAL RETARDATION

Parents may also find some of the magazines on the subject helpful. *Exceptional Parent* frequently has practical articles useful to parents of children with mental retardation. The address for subscription information is: P.O. Box 3000, Dept EP, Denville, NJ 07834-9919 (800-247-8080).

Parents seeking information on early intervention programs in their community should call their school district, state department of education office, or the local United Way office. If information is not available through these sources, the constituent service staff of state senators or representatives, county legislators, or city council members are often helpful. Telephone numbers and office locations for constituent service staff usually can be found in the telephone book, or through the reference desk at the public library.

Parents who are interested in joining advocacy and support groups may be interested in the following organizations:

The ARC — formerly the Association for Retarded Citizens of the United States. This is a national organization of parents, professionals, and advocates concerned about the needs of children and adults with mental retardation. Their address is 2501 Avenue J, P.O. Box 6109, Arlington, TX 76005 (817-640-0204). There are also many local offices and branches of the ARC. Check your telephone book or call the national office.

TASH — The Association for Persons with Severe Handicaps. This is also a national organization of parents, professionals, and advocates who are primarily concerned with the needs of children and adults with severe handicaps, including mental retardation. TASH also has a national headquarters and local chapters. The address of the national office is: 7010 Roosevelt Way, N.E., Seattle, WA 98115.

The National Down Syndrome Congress (NDSC) is also a valuable resource. Their address is 1800 Dempster Street, Park Ridge, IL 6008-1146 (800-232-6372).

Chapter 3

Much of the information in this chapter was obtained from the *News Digest* of the National Information Center for Children and Youth with Disabilities (NICHCY) in Washington, D.C. Parents

Recommended Resources | 253

may find NICHCY publications helpful. Their address is P.O. Box 1492, Washington, D.C. 20013 (800/999-5599).

A good book on the topic of special education and the appeals process is *Negotiating the Special Education Maze: A Guide for Parents and Teachers,* W. Anderson, S. Chitwood, and D. Hayden (Rockville, MD: Woodbine House, 1990).

Many state departments of education have guidebooks to the special education system for parents, and these guidebooks generally have a good comprehensive overview of special education in that state and include information on the appeals process for parents. The guidebooks are usually free and can be obtained through a local school district or library, or from the headquarters of your state department of education. Special education staff, including teachers, administrators, social workers, and others can also be good sources of information.

The following sources of information may also be of help to parents:

Baker and Brightman, *Steps to Independence.*

T. H. Powell and P. A. Ogle, *Brothers and Sisters — A Special Part of Exceptional Families.* Baltimore, MD: Brookes Publishing, 1985.

H. R. Turnbull, III, A. P. Turnbull, G. J. Bronicki, J. A. Summers, and C. Roeder-Gordon, *Disability and the Family.* Baltimore, MD: Brookes Publishing, 1989. An excellent guide for families preparing a teenager with mental retardation for adult life. Covers all of the important issues with a clear focus on practical topics and activities. A very good list of resources and references.

Chapter 5

Parents of adults with mental retardation have fewer resources available in many areas. The following books may be helpful:

Disability and the Family (1989).

Brothers and Sisters — A Special Part of Exceptional Families (1985).

Parts of the *Steps to Independence* book may also be relevant to families who need to do skills training with adults with mental retardation at home.

254 | THE GUIDE TO MENTAL RETARDATION

Chapter 6

The following resources may be helpful for the reader interested in seniors with mental retardation:

M. Stroud and E. Sutton, *Expanding Options for Older Adults with Developmental Disabilities: A Practical Guide to Achieving Community Access.* Baltimore, MD: Brookes Publishing, 1988.

M. Stroud and E. Sutton, *Activities Handbook and Instructor's Guide for Expanding Options for Older Adults with Developmental Disabilities.* Baltimore, MD: Brookes Publishing, 1988.

R. E. Edgerton and M. A. Gaston, *"I've Seen It All!" Lives of Older Persons with Mental Retardation in the Community.* Baltimore, MD: Brookes Publishing, 1991.

Notes on Individuals Interviewed

The author wishes to thank the following people, whose observations have been incorporated into this book.

Marcene Basch Johnson is Director of Education Services at the Brookside School, run by Ulster Association for Retarded Citizens, in Cottekill, New York.

Judy Capurso is Program Coordinator for UARC, Senior Program, Kingston, New York.

Rosalie Charpentier is a legal professional and an advocate for developmentally disabled individuals working for Mid-Hudson Legal Services, Poughkeepsie, New York.

Michaela D'Aquanni is a special education teacher in LaGrange, New York.

Gail Cohen is Coordinator of Early Intervention Services at the Brookside School, Cottekill, New York.

Dan Forte is Assistant Program Director at UARC Day Treatment Program, Kingston, New York.

Don Fraser is Case Manager at UARC Day Treatment Program, Kingston, New York.

John Gerdtz is Associate Professor of Psychiatry and Social Services, Emory University School of Medicine, Atlanta, Georgia.

THE GUIDE TO MENTAL RETARDATION

Mike Kessler, a teacher, administered early childhood and Head Start programs. He resides in La Grange, New York.
Bonnie Lester is a school psychologist in Kingston, New York.

Judy Livoti is Program Director, UARC Day Treatment program, Kingston, New York.

Al Marotta is a parent of a child with Down syndrome. He lives in Hopewell Junction, New York.

John Mordock is a psychologist who has worked with and written about individuals with mental retardation. He authored *The Other Children.*

Peter Pierri is Executive Director of Ulster ARC in Kingston, New York.

Don Rogers is a Trainer at UARC, Kingston, New York.

Jackie Romano is Director of Education and Training, UARC, Kingston, New York.

Without their help, this book would not have been possible.

Bibliography

Abramson, P. R., Parker, T., and Weisberg, S. R. (1988). Sexual Expression of Mentally Retarded People: Educational and Legal Implications. *American Journal on Mental Retardation,* 93: 328–334. American Association on Mental Retardation.

Ault, M. J., Wolery, M., Doyle, P. M., and Gast, D. L. (1989). Review of Comparative Studies in the Instruction of Students with Moderate and Severe Handicaps. *Exceptional Children,* 55: 346–356.

Baker, B. L. (1989). *Parent Training and Developmental Disabilities* (Monographs of the American Association on Mental Retardation, 13). Washington, DC: American Association on Mental Retardation.

Baker, B. L., and Brightman, A. J. (1989). *Steps to Independence. A Skills Training Guide for Parents and Teachers of Children with Special Needs.* Baltimore: Brookes Publishing.

Barcikowska, M., Silverman, W., Zigman, W., Kozlowski, P. B., Kujawa, M., Rudelli, R., and Wisniewski, H. M. (1989). Alzheimer-Type Neuropathology and Clinical Symptoms of Dementia in Mentally Retarded People without Down Syndrome. *American Journal on Mental Retardation,* 93: 551–557. American Association on Mental Retardation.

Begun, A. L. (1989). Sibling Relationships Involving Developmentally Disabled People. *American Journal on Mental Retardation,* 93: 566–574. American Association on Mental Retardation.

Benson, A. and Turnbull (1986). Changing Second Graders' Attitudes Toward People with Mental Retardation: Using Kid Power. *Mental Retardation,* 24, 44–45.

Benson, B. A. (1986). Anger Management Training. *Psychiatric Aspects of Mental Retardation Reviews,* 5: 51–56.

Braddock, D. (1987). *Federal Policy Toward Mental Retardation and Developmental Disabilities.* Baltimore: Brookes Publishing.

Bregman, J. D. and Hodapp, R. M. (1991). Current Developments in the Understanding of Mental Retardation. Part 1: Biological and Phenomenological Perspectives. *Journal of the American Academy of Child and Adolescent Psychiatry,* 30: 707–719.

Bregman, S. (1985). Assertiveness Training for Mentally Retarded Adults. *Psychiatric Aspects of Mental Retardation Reviews,* 4: 43–47.

258 | THE GUIDE TO MENTAL RETARDATION

Bromley, B. and Blacker, J. (1989). Factors Delaying Out-of-Home Placement of Children with Severe Handicaps. *American Journal of Mental Retardation,* 94: 284–291. American Association on Mental Retardation.

Brown, F. and Lehr, D. H. (1989). *Persons with Profound Disabilities: Issues and Practices.* Baltimore: Brookes Publishing.

Brown, L., Halpern, A. S., Hasazi, S. B., and Wehman, P. (1987). From School to Adult Living: A Forum on Issues and Trends. *Exceptional Children,* 53: 546–554. The Council for Exceptional Children.

Brown, L., Long, E., Udvari-Solner, A., Davis, L., Van Deventer, P., Ahlgren, D., Johnson, F., Gruenwald, L., and Jorgenson, J. (1989). The Home School: Why Students with Severe Disabilities must Attend the Schools of Their Brothers, Sisters, Friends, and Neighbors. *TASH,* 14 (1): 1–7.

Burleigh, M. (1990, February). Euthanasia and the Third Reich. *History Today,* pp. 11–16.

Burleigh, M. (1991). Euthanasia in the Third Reich: Some Recent Literature. *Social History of Medicine,* 4, 317–328.

Caruso, D. R. and Hodapp, R. M. (1988). Perceptions of Mental Retardation and Mental Illness. *American Journal on Mental Retardation,* 95: 118–124. American Association on Mental Retardation.

Castles, E. E. and Glass, C. R. (1986). Training in Social and Interpersonal Problem-Solving Skills for Mildly and Moderately Mentally Retarded Adults. *American Journal of Mental Deficiency,* 91: 35–42. American Association on Mental Deficiency.

Center for Developmental Disabilities (1987). *Best Practice Guidelines for Students with Intensive Educational Needs.* Burlington, VT: University of Vermont.

Clark, M. and Knowlton, J. (1987). Educational Technology and Children with Moderate Learning Difficulties. *Exceptional Child,* 33, 28–34.

Clegg, J. A. and Standen, P. J. (1991). Friendship among Adults Who Have Developmental Disabilities. *American Journal on Mental Retardation,* 95: 663–671. American Association on Mental Retardation.

Coates, D. (1988). Modification of Maternal Behavior in Efforts to Reduce Infant Mortality and Childhood Morbidity Associated with Low Birth Weight. In J. F. Kavanagh (ed.), *Understanding Mental Retardation: Research Accomplishments and New Frontiers.* Baltimore: Brookes Publishing, 105–136.

Cohen, D. J. and Bregman, J. D. (1988). Mental Disorders and Psychopharmacology of Retarded Persons: Another Step in Seeing the Whole Person. In J. F. Kavanagh (ed.) *Understanding Mental Retardation: Research Accomplishments and New Frontiers,* Baltimore: Brookes Publishing, 319–330.

Cohen, S. S. (1989) He's Not Broken. *Woman's Day,* 90–93.

Cole, C. L. and Gardner, W. I. (1984). Self-Management Training. *Psychiatric Aspects of Mental Retardation Reviews,* 3: 18–20.

Cole, D. A. and Meyer, L. H. (1989). Impact Needs and Resources on Family Plans to Seek Out-of-Home Placement. *American Journal on Mental Retardation,* 93: 380–387. American Association on Mental Retardation.

Cooke, R. E. (1988). Overview. In J. F. Kavanagh (ed.), *Understanding Mental Retardation: Research Accomplishments and New Frontiers,* Baltimore: Brookes Publishing, 291–296.

Bibliography | 259

Deutsch, H. (1985). Grief Counseling with the Mentally Retarded Clients. *Psychiatric Aspects of Mental Retardation Reviews,* 4: 17–20.

Deutsch, H. (1989). Stress, Psychological Defense Mechanisms, and the Private World of the Mentally Retarded: Applying Psychotherapeutic Concepts to Habilitation. *Psychiatric Aspects of Mental Retardation Reviews,* 8: 25–32.

DiFrancesco, P. J. (1989). Each Belongs: Educating All Children Together. Second Annual Conference sponsored by the Parent and Professional Special Education Advisory Council. Ontario, Canada.

Dunst, C. J., Trivette, C., and Deal, A. (1988). *Enabling and Empowering Families. Principles and Guidelines for Practice.* Cambridge, MA: Brookline Books.

Edgerton, R. B. (1979). *Mental Retardation.* Cambridge, MA: Harvard University Press.

Edgerton, R. B. (1988). Aging in the Community — A Matter of Choice. *American Journal on Mental Retardation,* 92: 331–335. American Association for Mental Retardation.

Education for All Handicapped Act of 1975, 612, 20 U.S.C. 1412.

Emerson, E. B. (1985). Evaluating the Impact of Deinstitutionalization on the Lives of Mentally Retarded People. *American Journal of Mental Deficiency,* 90: 277–288. American Association on Mental Deficiency.

Eyman, R. K., Call, T. I., and White, J. F. (1991). Life Expectancy of Persons with Down Syndrome. *American Journal on Mental Retardation,* 95: 603–612. American Association on Mental Retardation.

Fantuzzo, J. W., Wray, L. W., Hall, R., Goins, C., and Azar, S. (1986). Parent and Social-Skills Training for Mentally Retarded Mothers Identified as Child Maltreaters. *American Journal of Mental Deficiency,* 91: 135–140. American Association on Mental Deficiency.

Farber, B. (1986). Historical Contexts of Research on Families with Mentally Retarded Members. In J. J. Gallagher and P. M. Vietze (eds.), *Families of Handicapped Persons. Research, Programs, and Policy Issues.* Baltimore: Brookes Publishing.

Florian, L. D. and West, J. (1989). Congress Affirms the Rights of Children with Handicaps. *Teaching Exceptional Children,* 21 (4): 4–7.

Foxx, R. M., McMorrow, M. J., Storey, K., and Rogers, B. M. (1984). Teaching Social/Sexual Skills to Mentally Retarded Adults. *American Journal of Mental Deficiency,* 89, 9–15.

Fuchs, L. S., Fuchs, D., and Stecker, P. M. (1989). Effects of Curriculum-Based Measurement on Teachers' Instructional Planning. *Journal of Learning Disabilities,* 22 (1): 51–59.

Galler, J. R. (1988). Intergenerational Effects of Undernutrition. In J. F. Kavanagh (ed.), *Understanding Mental Retardation: Research Accomplishments and New Frontiers.* Baltimore: Brookes Publishing, 35–40.

Gerdtz, J. and Bregman, J. (1990). *Autism: A Practical Guide for Those Who Help Others.* New York: Continuum.

Gilson, S. F. and Levitas, A. S. (1987). Psychosocial Crisis in the Lives of Mentally Retarded People. *Psychiatric Aspects of Mental Retardation Reviews,* 6: 27–31.

Goldberg, S. S. and Kuriloff, P. J. (1991). Evaluating the Fairness of Special Education Hearings. *Exceptional Children,* 57: 546-555.

260 | THE GUIDE TO MENTAL RETARDATION

Grant, G. and McGrath, M. (1990). Need for Respite-Care Services for Caregivers of Persons with Mental Retardation. *American Journal on Mental Retardation*, 94: 638–648. American Association on Mental Retardation.

Griffiths, D. (1990a). Teaching Social Competency Part 1: Practical Guidelines. *The Habilitative Mental Healthcare Newsletter*, 9: 1–8.

Griffiths, D. (1990b). Teaching Social Competency Part 2: The Social Life Game. *The Habilitative Mental Healthcare Newsletter*, 9: 9–16.

Guralnick, M. J. (1991). The Next Decade of Research on the Effectiveness of Early Intervention. *Exceptional Children*, 58: 174–183.

Hanline, M. F. and Murray, C. (1984). Integrating Severely Handicapped Children into Regular Public Schools. *Phi Delta Kaplan*, 66: 273–276.

Haseltine, B. and Miltenberger, R. G. (1990). Teaching Self-Protection Skills to Persons with Mental Retardation. *American Journal on Mental Retardation*, 95: 188–197. American Association on Mental Retardation.

Haywood, H. C. (1988). Overview in J. F. Kavanagh (ed.), *Understanding Mental Retardation*. Baltimore: Brookes Publishing.

Hebbeler, K. M., Smith, B. J., and Black, T. (1991). Federal Early Childhood Special Education Policy: A Model for Improvement of Services for Children with Disabilities. *Exceptional Children*, 58: 104–112.

Heekin, S. (1984). New Friends. *Children Today*, 13: 8–13.

Helander, E. (1984). On Prejudice and Dignity. *World Health*, 18–19.

Heller, T. and Factor, A. (1991). Permanency Planning for Adults with Mental Retardation Living with Family Caregivers. *American Journal on Mental Retardation*, 96: 163–176. American Association on Mental Retardation.

Hentoff, N. (1983, December 13). The Baby Who Was Starved to Death for His Own Good. *Village Voice*, p. 6.

Hentoff, N. (1984, January 3). Troublemaking Babies and Pious Liberals. *Village Voice*, p. 8.

Hill, J. W., Seyfarth, J., Banks, P. D., Wehman, P., and Orelove, F. (1987). Parent Attitudes about Working Conditions of Their Adult Mentally Retarded Sons and Daughters. *Exceptional Children*, 54: 9–23. The Council for Exceptional Children.

Hill, M. L. (1988). Supported Competitive Employment: An Interagency Perspective. In P. Wehman and M. S. Moon (eds.), *Vocational Rehabilitation and Supported Employment*. Baltimore: Brookes Publishing, 31–54.

Hingsburger, D. (1987). Sex Counseling with the Developmentally Handicapped: The Assessment and Management of Seven Critical Problems. *Psychiatric Aspects of Mental Retardation Reviews*, 6: 41–46.

Hingsburger, D. (1988). Clients and Curriculum: Preparing for Sex Education. *Psychiatric Aspects of Mental Retardation Reviews*, 7: 13–18.

Hingsburger and Griffiths (1986). Dealing with Sexuality in a Community Residential Service. *Psychiatric Aspects of Mental Retardation Review*, 8: 63–68.

Hurley, A. D. and Sovner, R. (1986). Dementia, Mental Retardation, and Down Syndrome. *Psychiatric Aspects of Mental Retardation Reviews*, 5: 39–44.

Iverson, J. C. and Fox, R. A. (1989) Prevalence of Psychopathology among Mentally Retarded Adults.*Research in Developmental Disabilities,*10: 77–83.

Janicki, M. P. (1988). The Changing Nature of the Population with Mental Retardation: Historical Artifacts and Future Trends. *Mental Retardation Research*

Accomplishments and New Frontiers. Baltimore: Brookes Publishing, 297–310.

Johanson, C., Trivette, C., and Hamby, D. (1991). Family-Oriented Early Intervention Policies and Practices: Family-Centered or Not? *Exceptional Children,* 58: 115–126.

Kakalik, J. S., Furry, W. S., Thomas, M. A., and Carney, M. F. (1981). *The Cost of Special Education.* Santa Monica, CA: Rand Corporation.

Kanner, L. (1964). *A History of the Care and Study of the Mentally Retarded.* Springfield, IL: Charles C. Thomas.

Kavanagh, J. F. (ed.) (1988). *Understanding Mental Retardation: Research Accomplishments and New Frontiers.* Baltimore: Brookes Publishing.

Kelly, J. A. and Christoff, K. (1985). Job Interview Training. *Psychiatric Aspects of Mental Retardation Reviews,* 4: 5–8.

Koretz, G. (1992, February 10). High Taxes Are Not What's Ailing the U.S. Economy. *Business Week,* p. 20.

Krauss, M. W. (1988). Long-Term Care Issues in Mental Retardation. In J. F. Kavanagh (ed.), *Understanding Mental Retardation: Research Accomplishments and New Frontiers.* Baltimore: Brookes Publishing, 331–339.

Krauss, M. W. and Seltzer M. M. (1986). Comparison of Elderly and Adult Mentally Retarded Persons in Community and Institutional Settings. *American Journal of Mental Deficiency,* 91: 237–243. American Association on Mental Deficiency.

Levine, H. G. (1985). Situational Anxiety and Everyday Life Experiences of Mildly Mentally Retarded Adults. *American Journal of Mental Deficiency,* 90: 27–33. American Association on Mental Deficiency.

Lewin, Tamar (1990, October 28). As the Retarded Live Longer, Anxiety Grips Aging Parents. *The New York Times.*

Ludwig, S. and Hingsburger, D. (1989). Preparation for Counseling and Psychotherapy: Teaching about Feelings. *Psychiatric Aspects of Mental Retardation Reviews,* 8: 1-7.

Lyle, K. L. (1992, March 2). A Gentle Way to Die. *Newsweek,* p. 14.

Marston, D. (1988). Measuring Progress on IEPs: A Comparison of Graphing Approaches. *Exceptional Children,* 55, 38–44.

Matson, J. L. (1984). Social Skills Training. *Psychiatric Aspects of Mental Retardation Reviews,* 3: 1–4.

McLoughlin, C. S., Garner, J. B., and Callahan, M. (1987). *Getting Employed. Staying Employed.* Baltimore: Brookes Publishing.

McNergney, R. and Haberman, M. (1986). What Teaching Techniques Work Best with Mainstreamed Students? *NEA Today,* 4: 8.

Neubert, D. A., Tilson, Jr., G. P. and Ianacone, R. N. (1989). Postsecondary Transition Needs and Employment Patterns of Individuals with Mild Disabilities. *Exceptional Children,* 55: 494–500. The Council for Exceptional Children.

Neustadt, R. E., and May, E. R. (1986). *Thinking in Time. The Uses of History for Decision Makers.* New York: Free Press.

Nyhan, W. L. (1988). Research Challenges and Opportunities in the Next Quarter Century. In J. F. Kavanagh (ed.), *Understanding Mental Retardation. Research Accomplishments and New Frontiers.* Baltimore: Brookes Publishing, 3–18.

262 | THE GUIDE TO MENTAL RETARDATION

Patton, J., Payne, Bierne-Smith, M. (1986). *Mental Retardation.* 2nd ed. Columbus, OH: Merrill Publishing Co.

Pendler, B. and Hingsburger, D. (1990). Sexuality: Dealing with Parents. *The Habilitative Mental Healthcare Newsletter,* 9: 29–36.

Powell, T. H. and Ogle, P. A. (1985). *Brothers and Sisters — A Special Part of Exceptional Families.* Baltimore: Brookes Publishing.

Reiss, S. and Benson, B. A. (1985). Psychosocial Correlates of Depression in Mentally Retarded Adults: I. Minimal Social Support and Stigmatization. *American Journal of Mental Deficiency,* 89: 331–337. American Association on Mental Deficiency.

Richardson, S. A., Kuller, H., and Katz, M. (1988). Job Histories in Open Employment of a Population of Young Adults with Mental Retardation: I. *American Journal on Mental Retardation,* 92: 483–491. American Association on Mental Retardation.

Robinson, D., Griffith, J., McComish, K., and Swasbrook, K. (1984). Bus Training for Developmentally Disabled Adults. *American Journal of Mental Deficiency,* 89: 37–43. American Association on Mental Deficiency.

Schaffner, B., Buswell, B., Summerfield, A., Kovar, G., and Martz, J. (1988). *Discover the Possibilities: A Curriculum for Teaching Parents about Integration.* Peek Parent Center: Colorado Springs, Colorado.

Schalock, R. L. (1983). *Services for Developmentally Disabled Adults: Development, Implementation and Evaluation.* Baltimore: University Park Press.

Schalock, R. L. McGaughey, M. J., and Kiernan, W. E. (1989). Placement into Nonsheltered Employment: Findings from National Employment Surveys. *American Journal on Mental Retardation,* 94: 80–87. American Association on Mental Retardation.

Scheerenberger, R. C. (1983). *A History of Mental Retardation.* Baltimore,: Brookes Publishing.

Scheerenberger, R. C. (1987). *A History of Mental Retardation. A Quarter Century of Promise.* Baltimore: Brookes Publishing.

Schloss, P. J., Wolf, C. W., and Schloss, C. N. (1987). Financial Implications of Half- and Full-Time Employment for Persons with Disabilities. *Exceptional Children,* 54: 272–276. The Council for Exceptional Children.

Schulz, J. (1985). Growing Up Together. In J. R. Turnbull, III, and A. P. Turnbull (eds.) *Parents Speak Out: Then and Now.* Columbus, OH: Merrill, 11–20.

Seltzer, M. M. (1985). Informal Supports for Aging Mentally Retarded Persons. *American Journal of Mental Deficiency,* 90: 259–265. American Association on Mental Deficiency.

Seltzer, M. M. and Krauss, M. W. (1989). Aging Parents with Adult Mentally Retarded Children: Family Risk Factors and Sources of Support. *American Journal on Mental Retardation,* 94: 303–312. American Association on Mental Retardation.

Seltzer, M. M. and Krauss, M. W. (1987). *Aging and Mental Retardation.* Washington: American Association on Mental Retardation.

Sengstock, W. L., Magerhans-Hurley, and Sprotte, A. (1990 a) Germany, Cradle of American Special Education for Persons Who Are Mentally Retarded. *Education and Training in Mental Retardation,* 25: 4–14.

Bibliography | 263

Sengstock, W. L., Magerhans-Hurley, and Sprotte, A. (1990 b) The Role of Special Education in the Third Reich. *Education and Training in Mental Retardation*, 25: 225–236.

Shapira, Z., Cnaan, R. A., and Cnaan, A. (1985). Mentally Retarded Workers' Reactions to Their Jobs. *American Journal of Mental Deficiency*, 90: 160–166. American Association on Mental Deficiency.

Sherman, B. R. (1988). Predictors of the Decision to Place Developmentally Disabled Family Members in Residential Care. *American Journal on Mental Retardation*, 92: 344–351. American Association on Mental Retardation.

Shore, M. F., Brice, P. J., and Love, B. G. (1992). *When Your Child Needs Testing*. New York: Crossroad.

Staff (1987, August). Setting Up for a Special Student. *Instructor*, 97: 60–63.

Stahlman, M. T., Grogaard, J., Lindstrom, D. P., Haywood, N., and Culley, B. (1988). Neonatal Intensive Care and Developmental Outcome. In J. F. Kavanagh (ed.), *Understanding Mental Retardation: Research Accomplishments and New Frontiers*. Baltimore: Brookes Publishing, 171–178.

Stark, E. (1983). Disabilities, Puppets, and Play. *Psychology Today*, 17: 14–15.

Stoneman, Z. and Crapps, J. M. (1988). Mentally Retarded Individuals in Family Care Homes: Relationship with the Family of Origin. *American Journal on Mental Retardation*, 94: 420–430. American Association on Mental Retardation.

Storey, K. and Rogers, B. M. (1984). Teaching Social/Sexual Skills to Mentally Retarded Adults. *American Journal of Mental Deficiency*, 89: 9–15. American Association on Mental Deficiency.

Strain, P. S. (1988). *LRE for Preschool Children with Handicaps: What We Know, What We Should Be Doing*. Pittsburgh: Western Psychiatric Institute and Clinic.

Summers, J. A., Behr, S. K., and Turnbull, A. P. (1989) Positive Adaption and Coping Strengths of Families Who Have Children with Disabilities. In G. H. S. Singer and L. K. Irvin (eds), *Support for Caregiving Families*. Baltimore: Brookes Publishing, 27–40.

Szymanski, L. S. and Biederman, J. (1984). Depression and Anorexia Nervosa with Down Syndrome. *American Journal of Mental Deficiency*, 89: 246–251. American Association on Mental Deficiency.

Trach, J. S. and Rusch, F. R. (1989). Supportive Employment Program Evaluation: Evaluating Degree of Implementation and Selected Outcomes. *American Journal on Mental Retardation*, 94: 131–140. American Association on Mental Retardation.

Turkington, C. (1987). Special Talents: For Years Down Syndrome Was Another Name for Profound Mental Retardation and a One-Way Ticket to an Institution. *Psychology Today*, 21: 42–46.

Turnbull, III, H. R. and Turnbull, A. P. (1990). *Families, Professionals, and Exceptionality: A Special Partnership*. Columbus, OH: Merrill.

UNESCO (1987). Society and the Disabled. *UNESCO*, 29.

Valenti-Hein, D. C. (1990). A Dating Skills Program for Adults with Mental Retardation. *The Habilitative Mental Healthcare Newsletter*, 9: 47–54.

264 | THE GUIDE TO MENTAL RETARDATION

Waters, D., (1984). The Ten Commandments of Integrated Living. *World Health,* 23.

Woo, S. L. C. (1988). Molecular Biology: Phenylketonuria as a Model. In J. F. Kavanagh (ed.), *Understanding Mental Retardation: Research Accomplishments and New Frontiers.* Baltimore: Brookes Publishing, 41–56.

World Health. (1984). Togetherness Works. *World Health,* 19.

Zetlin, A. G. (1986). Mentally Retarded Adults and Their Siblings. *American Journal on Mental Deficiency,* 91: 217–225. American Association on Mental Deficiency.

Zetlin, A. G., and Turner, J. L. (1985). Transition from Adolescence to Adulthood: Perspectives of Mentally Retarded Individuals and their families. *American Journal of Mental Deficiency,* 89: 570–579. American Association on Mental Deficiency.

Zigler, E., Hodapp, R. M., and Edison, M. R. (1990). From Theory to Practice in the Care and Education of Mentally Retarded Individuals. *American Journal on Mental Retardation,* 95: 1–12. American Association on Mental Retardation.

Zigman, W. B., Schuff, N., Lubin, R. A., and Silverman, W. P. (1987). Premature Regression of Adults with Down Syndrome. *American Journal of Mental Deficiency,* 92: 161–168. American Association on Mental Deficiency.

Zigmond, N., and Miller, S. E. (1986). Assessment for Instructional Planning. *Exceptional Children,* 52: 501–509.

Glossary

AAMR   American Association on Mental Retardation

ARC   Association for Retarded Citizens

BOCES   Board of Cooperative Education Services

DDSO   Developmental Disabilities Service Office

DSS   Department of Social Services

EAHCA   Education for All Handicapped Children Act

EHA   Education of the Handicapped Act

HCPA   Handicapped Children's Protection Act of 1986

HRC   Human Rights Committee

ICF   Intermediate Care Facility

IDEA   Individuals with Disabilities Education Act

IEP   Individualized Education Program

ITT   Interdisciplinary Treatment Team

LRE   Least Restrictive Environment

NDSC   National Down Syndrome Congress

266 | THE GUIDE TO MENTAL RETARDATION

NICHCY   National Information Center for Children and Youth with Disabilities

OMRDD   Office of Mental Retardation and Developmental Disabilities

OSERS   Office of Special Education and Rehabilitation Services

TASH   The Association for Persons with Severe Handicaps

UCP   United Cerebral Palsy

WAC   Work Activities Center

WIC   Supplemental Food Program for Women, Infants, and Children